Decision Support Systems for Tele-medicine Applications

CSI: CONTROL AND SIGNAL/IMAGE PROCESSING SERIES

Series Editor: **Dr Peter A. Cook**
Control Systems Centre, UMIST, UK

1. Stabilisation of Nonlinear Systems: the piecewise linear approach
   Christos A. Yfoulis

2. Intelligent Systems - Fusion, Tracking and Control
   GeeWah Ng

3. Neural Network Control: Theory and Applications
   Sunan Huang, Kok Kiong Tan, Kok Zuea Tang

4. Decision Support Systems for Tele-medicine Applications
   George-Peter K. Economou

Decision Support Systems for Tele-medicine Applications

George - Peter K. Economou,
Electrical and Computer Engineer

(in collaboration with Phil Sotiriades, Physicist)

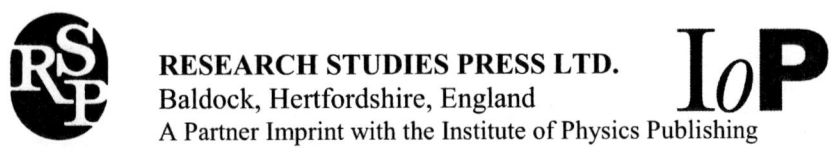

RESEARCH STUDIES PRESS LTD.
Baldock, Hertfordshire, England
A Partner Imprint with the Institute of Physics Publishing

RESEARCH STUDIES PRESS LTD.
16 Coach House Cloisters, 10 Hitchin Street, Baldock, Hertfordshire, SG7 6AE, England
Tel: + 44 (0)1462 895060, Fax: + 44 (0)1462 892546, E-mail: rsp@rspltd.demon.co.uk;
www.research-studies-press.co.uk

and

Institute *of* **Physics** PUBLISHING, Suite 929, The Public Ledger Building,
150 South Independence Mall West, Philadelphia, PA 19106, USA

Copyright © 2004, by **Research Studies Press** Ltd.
Research Studies Press Ltd. is a partner imprint with the Institute *of* **Physics** PUBLISHING

All rights reserved.
No part of this book may be reproduced by any means, nor transmitted, nor translated
into a machine language without the written permission of the publisher.

Marketing:

Institute *of* **Physics** PUBLISHING, Dirac House, Temple Back, Bristol, BS1 6BE, England
www.bookmarkphysics.iop.org

Distribution:

NORTH AMERICA
AIDC, 50 Winter Sport Lane, PO Box 20, Williston, VT 05495-0020, USA
Tel: 1-800 632 0880 or outside USA 1-802 862 0095, Fax: 802 864 7626, E-mail: orders@aidcvt.com

UK AND THE REST OF WORLD
Marston Book Services Ltd, P.O. Box 269, Abingdon, Oxfordshire, OX14 4YN, England
Tel: + 44 (0)1235 465500, Fax: + 44 (0)1235 465555, E-mail: direct.order@marston.co.uk

Library of Congress Cataloging-in-Publication Data

Economou, George-Peter K., 1966-
 Decision support systems for tele-medicine applications / George-Peter K. Economou, in
collaboration with Phil Sotiriades.
    p. cm. -- (Csi, control and signal/image processing series)
 Includes bibliographical references and index.
 ISBN 0-86380-287-7
 1. Medical telematics. 2. Decision support systems. 3. Expert systems (Computer science)
4. Neural networks (Computer science) I. Sotiriades, Phil. II. Title. III. Series.
 R119.95.E27 2004
 610'.285--dc22
                              2004007498

British Library Cataloguing in Publication Data
A catalogue record for this book is available from the British Library.

ISBN 0 86380 287 7

Printed in Great Britain by Lighnting Source. Cover artwork by Brookhill Design
Studio.

Editorial Foreword

This new series of books had its origin in the UMIST Control Systems Centre Series, previously edited by my colleagues Professor Peter Wellstead and Dr Martin Zarrop, which concentrated on making widely and rapidly available the results of research undertaken in the Centre. The aim of the new series, while continuing to concentrate on the areas of Control and Signal/Image Processing, is to provide a wider channel of publication for any author who have novel and important research results, or critical surveys of particular topics, to communicate. My hope and intention is that the series will offer an interesting and useful resource to research workers, students and academics in the fields covered, as well as appealing to the engineering community in general.

The present volume constitutes something of a departure from the main thrust of the CSI series, but is nevertheless appropriate to it, partly because decision support systems (DSSs) have already attracted the attention of control engineers, and also because the methodology employed here is based on artificial neural networks (ANNs), which have been fundamental to the two immediately preceding books in the series. Being concerned with diagnosis, this medical decision support system (MDSS) presents a new methodology for producing Learning Patterns and also contributes to the application of engineering concepts in the life sciences; consequently lies in an area which is certain to become increasingly important as biological issues achieve greater prominence in the public mind. It is a distinctive work, largely the product of the author's personal endeavours in the Tele-medicine field, which I hope and expect will obtain wide appreciation as a result of its publication.

Peter Cook

Control Systems Centre
Department of Electrical Engineering & Electronics
UMIST, Manchester, United Kingdom

Preface

by Dr. George - Peter K. Economou

A novel decision support system with modular structure is proposed, developed on the basis of artificial neural networks (ANNs) and applied to research areas where human experience is employed for the promotion of decisions. The architecture of this system can be adapted to the existing structures of the application field and is arranged according to the classification of the input data. The data provided are exactly in the form an expert would operate on them. The hierarchical structure with which the system processes the input data calls for intermediate decisions, and promotes the final decision from the general to the more specific classes in which the area of interest can be divided. The system's operation eventually prompts for new data to be fed.

These new inputs are supplied to the system in succeeding processing levels, while time as a discriminating factor for some of the previously input data is being accounted for. The implemented system is input data that have not undergone pre-processing or symbolic restructuring.

This system was adapted and thoroughly tested in the field of medicine with very good results. Because of the incomplete inputs of this area, a new representation of the learning patterns (used for teaching its ANNs) was created and hereby demonstrated. This representation can be generally arranged during the learning procedure of ANNs and its main characteristic consists of manipulating incomplete input data for the teaching, testing, and employment of these networks. The data components are inserted separately; their particular value is enhanced and pseudo-inputs are set during the ANNs' learning procedure, smoothing their classification into different output classes. Previous research efforts simply ignored those data or filled them statistically. In addition, the number of hidden layers and artificial neurons were investigated as a factor affecting the performance of ANNs, as well as the importance of ANNs' weights. As a consequence, heuristic rules are suggested that consider the specification of ANNs values and intervene to change them before and after the networks' convergence.

Moreover, an architecture is proposed for the implementation of the new system in hardware. The feed-forward ANN's artificial neurons are approximated and circuits for their integration on silicon wafers are presented. They cover a large spectrum of specifications, offering some advantages like the re-targeting of the system's implementation in hardware, a generic development platform, independence from the manufacturer and from the utilized CAD tool.

Preface

by Dr. Phil Sotiriades

Back in February 2000, I began my Ph.D. research work that was to explore the field of developing new Tele-Working Protocols and applications. My dissertation also aimed to the dissemination of the Tele-Working Services and their benefits, by the utilization of Distributed Computing Systems.

By that time I met Dr. Economou who was working in the Tele-Medicine field. His work was complementary to mine and that led us to start a common project on how to exploit Tele-Working as a means to diffuse his MDSS. I have reason to believe this book will not be the only one to bear our results.

Working to establish Tele-Working protocols in no easy task. "Tele-Working", both as a meaning and as a tool can be regarded both psychologically (i.e. how to manage to deal with the everyday job's tasks while being at home) and technologically (i.e. what to conceive/build/standardize so to reach a means that should allow someone to remotely access his/her office's facilities).

However, international R&D projects seem to agree that Tele-Work should offer a platform for a variety of operations (i.e. electronic data interchange, audio/visual interface implementation, processing speed, etc.). Thus, the International Telecommunication Union produced standards on different Tele-Working applications (such as Tele-Medicine or Tele-Education, even differentiating sub-services like Tele-Surgery), and not for a whole service.

Keeping that in mind, we first focused on Tele-Medicine as the main application. However, the areas we explored (and whose aspects are given in Chapter 6) can be more generally applied to other aspects of everyday life as well. After all, should a Tele-Medicine integral service be suitable for human care then it surely can be adapted to cover other activities as well...

Contents

List of Figures xii

List of Tables xiv

Glossary and Abbreviations xv

Studying the Book: Structure and Scope 1
Structure 1
Scope 2
References 2

1st Chapter
An Introduction to Artificial Neural Networks (ANNs)
1.1 Introduction to ANNs 5
1.2 Artificial Neural Networks' Elements 5
1.3 Artificial Neural Networks' Training 7
1.4 Artificial Neural Networks' Categories 8
1.5 Well Known Artificial Neural Networks 8
1.6 Artificial Neural Networks' Training Algorithms 10
1.7 The Back Propagation Training Rule 11
1.8 The Back Propagation Rule and Kalman Filtering 12
1.9 Artificial Neural Networks' Application Areas 14
1.10 Artificial Neural Networks in Hardware 14
1.11 Artificial Neural Networks' Advantages 14
1.12 Conclusion 16
1.13 References 16

2nd Chapter
Decision Support Systems
2.1 Introduction 19
2.2 Necessity for Structuring Decision Support Systems 19
2.3 Decision Support Systems' Basic Structures 21
2.4 Decision Support Systems' Training 22
2.5 Decision Support Systems' Disadvantages 24
2.6 The Contribution of Artificial Neural Networks 25
2.7 The Basic Artificial Neural Network 27

2.8	Requirements for a Novel Decision Support System	27
2.9	The Novel Decision Support System	29
2.10	Comparison with the Adaptive Expert Network	31
2.11	Conclusion	33
2.12	References	34

3rd Chapter
Medical Decision Support Systems

3.1	Introduction	37
3.2	Decision Support Systems in Medicine	37
3.3	Medical Decision Support Systems' Specifications	39
	3.3.1 The Users' Demands	39
	3.3.2 Dynamics of Medical System's Development	39
	3.3.3 Results from the Use of Artificial Neural Networks	41
3.4	Brief Description of Previous Medical Systems	42
	3.4.1 Finding Elements Displaying the Existence of Gastric Cancer	42
	3.4.2 Finding Elements Displaying the Existence of Dementia	43
	3.4.3 Finding Elements Displaying the Existence of Hypertension	44
	3.4.4 Finding Elements Displaying a Distinction between Malignant Tumours	46
	3.4.5 Finding Elements Displaying the Existence of Malignant Melanoma	47
3.5	Conclusions Gathered from the Use of Previous Medical Systems	49
3.6	Clinical Differential Diagnosis Methodology	50
	3.6.1 Understanding of Medical Events	51
	3.6.2 Assessment of Medical Events	51
	3.6.3 Drawing Out a Series of Assumptions	51
	3.6.4 Selection between Assumptions	51
3.7	Medical Examination with the Novel Medical System	52
3.8	Application of the Novel Medical System in Pulmonology	53
	3.8.1 Grouping of Pulmonary Medical Data	53
	3.8.2 Architecture of the Pulmonary Medical System	56
	3.8.3 Control and Exploitation of the Pulmonary Medical System	61
3.9	Application of the Medical System in Haematology	64
	3.9.1 Grouping of Haematology Medical Data	64
	3.9.2 Architecture of the Haematology Medical System	65
	3.9.3 Control and Exploitation of the Haematology Medical System	65
3.10	Conclusions from Exploiting the Two Medical Systems	65
3.11	Specialized Uses of the Novel Medical System	66
3.12	Conclusions	67
3.13	References	67

4th Chapter
Artificial Neural Network Learning Procedure

4.1	Introduction	71
4.2	Forms of Learning Patterns	71

4.3	The Output-centred Learning Patterns' Form	74
4.4	The Proposed Input-centred Learning Patterns' Form	75
4.5	Application of the "Form-2" of the Learning Patterns	76
4.6	Assessment of the Hidden Neurons	84
4.7	The Synapses' Weights	85
4.8	Approximations for Less Hardware and Faster Convergence	87
4.9	Conclusions	94
4.10	References	95

5th Chapter
Implementation of the MDSS in Hardware

5.1	Introduction	97
5.2	The Implementation in Hardware	97
5.3	General Observations Concerning the Novel System	98
5.4	Approximation of the Artificial Neuron	98
5.5	Use of the Field Programmable Gate Arrays	100
5.6	Implementation's Structure	101
5.7	The Implemented Neuron	102
5.8	Neuron's Design	103
	5.8.1 The Proposed Multiplier-Adder/Accumulator	103
	5.8.2 Numerical Representation and Sigmoid	105
5.9	Implementation's Important Features	106
5.10	Definition of an Application's Parameters	107
5.11	A Comparison of the Novel Implementation's Traits	107
5.12	Parametrical Hardware Design	109
5.13	ANNs' Design using the VHDL Language	109
5.14	Conclusion	112
5.15	References	112

6th Chapter
Merging the DSS into a Tele-Working Platform

6.1	Introduction	115
6.2	Tele-Working Platform's General Characteristics	116
6.3	Two-tier Tele-Medicine Architecture	117
6.4	Transition from two-Tier to n-Tier Architecture	118
6.5	Interface Implementation	120
6.6	TWPL COM Components' Features	121
	6.6 1 TWPL Object vs Table	122
	6.6.2 Interface Definition Language and Globally Unique Identifiers	122
6.7	TWPL Components Activation	122
	6.7.1 Class Factories	123
	6.7.2 The IUnknown Interface	123
	6.7.3 Binding Technique	124
	6.7.4 Out-Of-Process Server	124
	6.7.5 Out-of-Process Activation	125
	6.7.6 Location Transparency Importance	126

6.8	Internet-based Tele-Medicine Service Applications	126
6.9	Conclusion	129
6.10	References	129

7th Chapter
Conclusions - Future Work
7.1	Conclusions	131
7.2	Future Work	133
7.3	References	134

| **Appendix I** | **The MDSS Demo** | 135 |
| Application | | 135 |

| **Appendix II** | **More on Type Libraries** | 139 |
| GUIDs | | 139 |

Appendix III	**COM/CORBA/XML & HTML**	141
COM		141
CORBA		141
XML & HTML		142

Index 143

List of Figures

1 Introduction
1.1 Structure of a Typical Artificial Neuron — 6
1.2 Feed-Forward Architecture (FFA) — 7

2 Decision Support Systems
2.1 Decision Support System — 21
2.2 Interaction during DSSs' Structuring — 22
2.3 The Novel Decision Support System — 29
2.4 A Section of Haykin's Adaptive Expert Network — 32

3 Medical Decision Support Systems
3.1 Architecture of the Novel Medical Decision Support System — 56
3.2 Schematic Representation of Layer #1 — 58

4 Artificial Neural Network Learning Procedure
4.1 Learning Patterns "Form-1" Input and Output Vectors — 73
4.2 Three Contrasted Learning Patterns "Form-1" Input Vectors — 74
4.3 Learning Patterns "Form-1" I/O Vectors — 76
4.4 Transformed input_vector_a (intermediate_form_1) — 77
4.5 Transformed input_vector_b (intermediate_form_1) — 78
4.6 Transformed input_vector_c (intermediate_form_1) — 79
4.7 Transformed input_vector_a (intermediate_form_2) — 80
4.8 Transformed input_vector_b (intermediate_form_2) — 81
4.9 Transformed input_vector_c (intermediate_form_2) — 82
4.10 Learning Patterns "Form-2" I/O Vectors — 83
4.11 Synapses' Weights (150th Cycle) — 88
4.12 Synapses' Weights (300th Cycle) — 88
4.13 Synapses' Weights (450th Cycle) — 89
4.14 Synapses' Weights (600th Cycle) — 89
4.15 Synapses' Weights (750th Cycle) — 90
4.16 Synapses' Weights (900th Cycle) — 90
4.17 Synapses' Weights (150th Cycle) — 91
4.18 Synapses' Weights (300th Cycle) — 91
4.19 Synapses' Weights (450th Cycle) — 92
4.20 Synapses' Weights (600th Cycle) — 92
4.21 Synapses' Weights (750th Cycle) — 93
4.22 Synapses' Weights (900th Cycle) — 93

5 Implementation of the MDSS in Hardware
5.1	The Two Sigmoid Functions	99
5.2	System's Units Connections	102
5.3	Implemented Neuron	103
5.4	The Proposed Multiplier - Adder/Accumulator	104
5.5	A 3-digit Number throughout the Multiplier - Adder/Accumulator	105
5.6	The Sigmoid Function's Approximation	105
5.7	FPGA's Contents	106
5.8	MDSS Updating Procedure Scheme	107
5.9	VHDL Behavioural Model of A Neuron (headers)	110
5.10	VHDL Behavioural Model of A Neuron (body)	111
5.11	Implemented VHDL Neuron Model	111

6 Integration of the MDMS into a Tele-Working Platform
6.1	Tele-Medicine Service Schematic Representation	116
6.2	Two-tier Application and Direct User's Connection to the Server	117
6.3	Two-tier Connections and Heterogeneous Data Sources	119
6.4	Introducing a Middle Layer of TWP Components	120
6.5	The Mapping between TWPL Components and Data Access Layer	121
6.6	A Proxy/Stub Layer	124
6.7	Inter-process Communication	127
6.8	TWPL, IIS, and HTML	128

Appendix I The MDSS Demo
I.1	MDSSs' Initial Medical Data Input Screen	135
I.2	Inputs for a Symptom's Sub-category	136
I.3	A Sub-diagnosis Resulted from Fig. I.2's Inputs	136
I.4	A Final Diagnosis Screen	137
I.5	Suggested Laboratory Examinations Screens	137

List of Tables

1 Introduction
   1.1   Well Known ANNs and their Characteristics   10

3 Medical Decision Support Systems
   3.1   Wheezing Findings per Category of Pulmonary Diseases   60
   3.2   Neurons and Synapses of Layer #1   62
   3.3   Neurons and Synapses of Layer #2   63
   3.4   Neurons and Synapses of Layer #3   64

Glossary and Abbreviations

Symbols
    .NET Framework - A platform for building, deploying, and running Web Services and applications (Microsoft technology).
    C - Software Programming Language

A
    ANN(s) - Artificial Neural Network(s)
    ASIC(s) - Application Specific Integrated Circuit(s)
    ASP - Active Server Pages
    ATM - Asynchronous Transfer Mode (tele-communication protocol)

B
    Bit(s) - Binary Digit(s)

C
    CLBs - Configurable Logic Block(s)
    CLSID - Class ID
    COM - Component Object Model (software design)
    CORBA - Common Object Request Broker Architecture

D
    DBMS(s) - Database Management System(s)
    DCOM - Distributed Component Object Model (software design)
    DCS - Distributed Computing System
    DTD - Document Type Definition
    DSS(s) - Decision Support System(s)

E
    Email - Electronic Mail (facilities)

F
    FFA - Feed Forward Architecture (ANN design)
    FPGA - Field Programmable Gate Array (hardware design)

G
    GUID(s) - Graphic User Interface(s)

H
H-MDSS - Haematology MDSS
HTML - Hypertext Markup Language

I
I/O - Input/Output
IEEE - Institute of Electrical and Electronic Engineers
IDL - Interface Definition Language
IID - Interface ID
IIS(s) - Internet Information Server(s)
ISDN - Integrated Services Digital Network (tele-communication protocol)
I-TWPL - (user-defined) Interface TWPL

J
JAVA - Software Programming Language

L
LAN - Local Area Network
Layer - Part of the (M)DSS (system design)
Level - Part of an ANN (ANN design)

M
MD(s) - Medical Doctor(s)
MDSS(s) - Medical Decision Support System(s)
Medical System(s) - Medical Decision Support System(s)
MS - Most Significant (digit -hardware design)
MS-Visual Basic - Software Programming Language
MS-Visual C++ - Software Programming Language
MUX - Multiplexer (hardware design)

O
ODBC - Open Database Connectivity (database communication protocol)
OMG - Object Management Group
ORB - Object Request Broker

R
R&D - Research and Development
RAM - Random Access Memory (hardware design)
RDBMS - Remote DBMS

S
SCM - Service Control Manager
Sigmoid - A Special-form Function (ANN design)
Slab - Part of an ANN (ANN design)
SQL - Structured Query Language (database design)
System(s) - Decision Support System(s)

T
    TLA - Three-Letter Acronym
    TMS(s) - Tele-Medicine Service(s)
    TWP(s) - Tele-Working Platform(s)
    TWPL - Tele-Working Platform addressing Layer

V
    VHDL - VLSI Hardware Description Language (hardware design)
    VLSI - Very Large Scale of Integration (hardware design)

W
    WAN - Wide Area Network

X
    XML - Extensible Markup Language

Studying the Book

Structure and Scope

Is there anything more interesting in life than searching for answers?
I. Asimov

Structure

This book is arranged in seven (7) chapters; therein the details of a Decision Support System (DSS) based on Artificial Neural Networks (ANNs) are presented. Moreover, the adaptations made for the system to cover a specific field (medicine) and a particular area (e.g. pulmonary diseases), and the course it undertook to be a part of a full-equipped Tele-Medicine platform are also given. The book concludes with the implementation details for the Tele-Medicine network structuring and specifically the use of DCOM and .NET facilities.

This Chapter offers an introduction of the books' chapters and presents its scope.

Chapter 1 can be described as an induction Chapter, where ANNs various elements, training methods, categories and algorithms are presented.

Chapter 2 shows the need to develop decision support systems. A brief introduction and the history of their evolution are also given, concluding with a presentation of medicine related DSSs. By means of a new model structure that is based on FFA-ANNs, a general system architecture is implemented which exploits the use of application structures that depend on human experience and expertise.

The novel system is implemented in the domain of medicine, as portrayed in Chapter 3. The relative bibliography is also analysed, the disadvantages of previous systems discussed, and the necessary explanation for the chosen evolutionary route for the new Medical Decision Support System (MDSS) is given.

The research results for the training procedure of our FFA-ANN - after extended analysis on those elements that are related to the neurons and synapses as well as with its weights - are shown in Chapter 4. A new mapping methodology of I/O data is recommended in order to form training patterns; the way of obtaining hidden neuron's number is studied and some heuristic methods for the intervention in a network's topology and weights after its convergence are proposed. Decrease in hardware use during the DSS implementation is studied, further improvements are specified and comparative results are pointed out.

The implementation of the above MDSS in hardware is the subject of Chapter 5. The architecture of the system and also the improvements and the differences in the topology of FFA-ANNs analysed. The presented implementation improves the speed of obtaining results and permits the adaptation of the implemented system in hardware to other application fields.

In Chapter 6, the novel DSS is adapted to be a part of a more general Tele-Working platform. Therefore, the hardware and software developing norms are described and real-world scenarios of its application are given. Also set are the operation of modern techniques and the use of DCOM and .NET facilities to structure, chart, and control the nodes of a whole Tele-Working service.

Conclusions about the system, its applications, and its possibilities of expansion in the future are the subjects of Chapter 7.

A great effort was made in this book to define the terminology before its use, with special care given to acronyms, since it spans a great variety of scientific areas. In this respect, the section with glossary and abbreviated terms should help even the most un-initiated reader. Finally, the reader has to keep in mind that this book represents well over twelve years of R&D from the part of the author.

Scope

The aim was to prepare a book intended for a variety of readers. The author wrote it with the general idea to address professionals in the areas of medicine, namely engineers, MDs, paramedics, people working on data information systems, and academic researchers. The proposed outcome of the book is a working Decision Support System (DSS) tested in a University Hospital's environment.

The book can be seen both from a professional trying to establish Tele-Working platforms, distant health care systems, etc., and a researcher's point of view. Moreover, it deals not only with the facets that set up this DSS, but also the collaboration principles that have to be established in order for so many experts (from so many different fields) to produce an outcome. Glossary, specifications, systems, and other problems are analysed step by step and proper solutions are proposed. The DSS's implementation in software and also in hardware are handled too [E95 I].

Many years of research were spent in setting up a general decision support system capable of being adapted to many fields of human expertise, its implementation specific to the field of medicine, and its progress thereafter. Thus, it includes previous attempts, results and experimental outcomes as well as medical data, symptoms' tables, diagnoses traits, etc., that were generated during those years [E95 II].

This book can also be a useful tool in a comparative survey of DSSs, expert systems advantage and disadvantages, ANNs, learning patterns generation, harware/software design of ANNs, etc. [E96]. On the other hand, topics about the way things are run in hospitals (e.g. patients' records, clinical differential diagnosis methodology, examination routines, etc.) are also covered in a way that computer engineers can readily utilize its data. All summed up, a book profitable to many readers.

References

[E95 I] Economou, G. - P., K., Hallas, J. A., Mariatos, E. P., and Goutis, C. E., "Artificial Neural Networks in Medical Decision Making Systems: An Application to Pulmonary Diseases' Diagnosis through VHDL Synthesis", Proc. of 1995 European Design and Test Conference & EuroASIC Exhibition, Paris, France, Mar. 1995.

[E95 II] Economou, G. - P. K., Economopoulos, N. M., Lymberopoulos, D., and C. E. Goutis, "Experiences Accumulated Working towards Medical

Decision Support Systems", J. of Microprocessing and Microprogramming, vol. 40, pp. 883-886, 1995.

[E96] Economou, G. - P. K., Goumas, P.D., and Spiropoulos, K., "A Novel Medical Decision Support System", IEE Computing & Control Engineering Journal, vol. 7, pp. 177 - 183, 1996.

4

1st Chapter

An Introduction to Artificial Neural Networks

The first step to the road to wisdom is the admittance of ignorance…
C. Giarrantano

1.1 Introduction

Artificial neural networks (ANNs) constitute a technological substitute to biological neural networks. These latter ones are the recognised keystones on which the superior functions of all beings are based; it is a well-known fact, also, that they designed to vary according to the specific application. ANNs are developed on a the basis of biological networks - in order to be studied - and at the same time they greatly model unknown characteristics of a target space's sampled data. As their response improves - as long as the samples of input/output data with whom they are "trained" increases - the networks "learn" and their operating mechanisms essentially back-up the experience that is inherent in these data [A&R88].

The mapping of an ANN's given inputs in wanted outputs (both generally given as vectors) is succeeded regardless of the many-to-choose network's alternatives (should input/output (I/O) data meet some rules), intensifying the search for the most efficient ANN (per given target space). Consequently, most researchers suggest their own exemplary ANN, that ensures different performance depending on the application and the specifications that must be fulfilled.

During the last decade, the use and research of ANNs was rekindled and resulted in viable solutions concerning multi-folded scientific and practical problems. In the mid '80s, researchers outweighed previous restrictions [M&P69] - developed by existing networks [A&R88] - and proposed others [H&H93]. The development of integrated electronic circuits has also given great impetus to the evolution of ANNs that have great demands in data memory. Their use has succeeded in the exploitation of networks' processing speed, a functional feature that is important for their chosen role.

1.2 Artificial Neural Networks' Elements

ANNs consist of networks of similar, or not, elements - the (artificial) **Neurons**. They vary in structure and function, as much as in their connections (called "**Synapses**"). Artificial neurons have been designed type, connection links, and functions that are in many ways similar to biological neurons. Fig. 1.1 shows a typical artificial neuron [McC43, Lip87].

The I/O data of a neuron generally obeys the following equation:

$$\psi = \varphi(\sum_{i=1}^{n} \beta_i * \chi_i) \qquad \text{(Equation 1.1)}$$

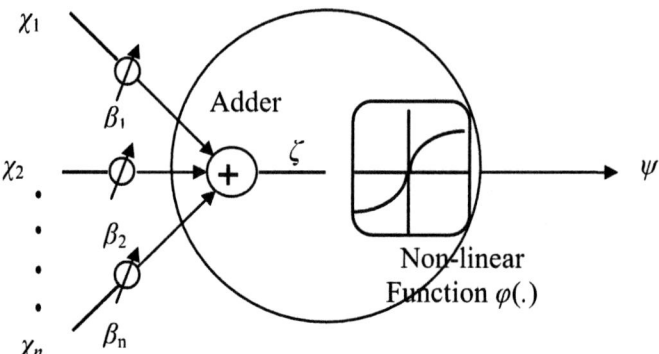

Figure 1.1: Structure of a Typical Artificial Neuron

A Neuron can accept large number of (digital or analog) inputs ($\chi_1, \chi_2, ..., \chi_n$), multiply them with the factors $\beta_1, \beta_2, ..., \beta_n$ (called "**Weights**"), and extract an output that can feed similar, or not, neurons. The outputs can be made discrete or analogue and when they have a non-zero value the neuron is said to have "**fired**". The weighed inputs sum up and are expressed in a non-linear function $\varphi(.)$.

Variations to the above structure are: neurons that insert the products of their input's combination [Vem88]; have their Weights mapped only in binary values (it can be considered as an attribute of a specific value to them) [H&H93]; develop totally different I/O relationships [RMS92].

The non-linear function $\varphi(.)$ corresponds to biological models' performance (capability for a neuron to fire), called "**Sigmoid**" (in honour of the Hellenic capital letter "Σ") and its typical forms can be [Lip87]:

$$\varphi(\zeta) = \text{sign}(\zeta), \varphi(\zeta) = \frac{1}{1+e^{-\zeta - \Pi}}, \varphi(\zeta) = \frac{1-e^{-\alpha * \zeta}}{1+e^{-\alpha * \zeta}}, \quad \text{(Equation 1.2)}$$

where "e" stands for the base of the natural (Napier) logarithms and the constants Π and α represent the slope of the Sigmoid function and a biased input, respectively. The last term forces the response of a neuron into a wanted value, given a certain input. The Sigmoid composes the non-linear term, which will play an important role in the input's **classification**, depending on the application. The bigger the slope, the less clear the limits of the classes that are defined [Lip87]. The choice of its form is related to both the application and the methodology on the basis of which the ANN shall relate inputs to output (during **training**).

Neurons can be connected in many ways, creating ANN **architectures** (e.g. as in Fig. 1.2). These connections greatly define the application, extensibility, functionality, accuracy, and complexity rate of the network. Fig. 1.2, presents the widely used feed-forward architecture (FFA) [Lip87].

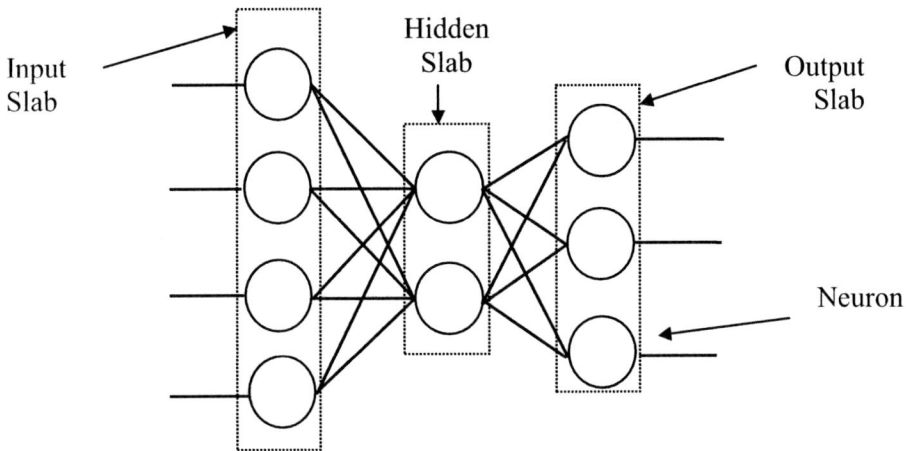

Figure 1.2: Feed-Forward Architecture (FFA)

In a FFA-ANN, the connections are only allowed in a single course between neuron "**Slabs**" (neurons belonging to the same architecture level). Between input and output Slabs and depending on the application, a number of **hidden** Slabs of neurons in which input vectors do not have immediate access and are not connected directly to the response of ANNs, intervene. The number of the hidden Slabs or/and neurons defines the behavioural performance and the effectiveness of FFA-ANNs.

1.3 Artificial Neural Networks' Training

For selecting an ANN capable to simulate the traits of a target space, the choice of its **Training Algorithm,** i.e. the methodology with which I/O data will result into proper weights in its Synapses, is most important. The algorithm can be part of a network's architecture, so dictating the neurons' connections [Hop82]. The procedure by which I/O data are made ready to be fed in ANNs is called "**mapping**".

During the application of a training algorithm, input- and output-**Patterns** (data) are fed into the Network that must adapt its Weights to make the inputs converge on the outputs, minus a pre-selected error threshold. This error is defined as the deviation of an ANN's pre-final convergence output from each output-pattern separately, based on whichever norm will be demanded from the user (i.e. the minimum, the mean square, etc. of all or individual outputs).

The Training Patterns must sufficiently represent the target space that they define. This space is approximated by the gradual learning of its subsections and an ANN should create a classification of the hyperspace those Patterns define, split in sections that must correspond in the most possible equal number of Patterns (equally distributed hyperspace). It depends on the user's choices if the ANN will **memorize** I/O pairs and simply will recall them or will **correlate** them, so as in the future to be able to furnish proper outputs that have not been given any enhanced characteristics.

During the training, the ANN's Weights readjust constantly so that from the input they process the wanted response is extracted (minus the training error).

In the case where the Networks are unable to respond correctly to a given input, they do not **converge** and cannot be trained, under the current methodology. A number of adjustments is then required, depending on the user's choices. For the FFA-ANN, augmentation of the number of the hidden Slabs/Neurons is often proposed [Lip87], tuning of the training parameters, etc. [§4.4|6|7|8].

1.4 Artificial Neural Networks' Categories

A maxim referring to the application field of ANNs defines them as approaches of the **optimum classifiers**. To that effect, most Networks are called to solve generalized or non- problems that are applied in classification. Thus, innumerable improvements to existing Neurons, ANNs' architectural, and their training algorithms are constantly being suggested. Despite the difficulties, the ANNs can be distributed in some general categories [W&L90]:

Continuous or **discrete**, depending on **time** considerations. Continuously operating Neurons produce partial outputs in different times than others, affecting a Network also during the transition of their outputs.

Analogue or **digital** depending on the implementation of their Neurons in **hardware**. The ANNs can also be emulated in software.

Operating to **float-** or **integer-** inputs and outputs, depending on the **numerical representation** of the components of their I/O vectors. Combinations in the utilization of those representations also comprise a valid choice.

Full- or **partially-** connected. Partially-connected Networks demand more advanced training algorithms but have less memory storage demands.

Supervised or **non-supervised**, depending on their **training algorithm**. The non-supervised ANNs converge to their outputs through processing their inputs intrinsic data that either are stored in or are detected by them.

Other categories of ANNs have been oriented in their matching fields - a detailed analysis of this topic is not within the scope of this book. Also, these Networks have a limited capability in evolving into new inputs and applications.

1.5 Well Known Artificial Neural Networks

The following description briefly covers the more frequently-used Artificial Neural Networks used to date. More details are given in [A&R88, F&S91, H&H93, Lip87, Pao89, Vem88, W&L90], where specialized forms are presented.

Adaptive Resonance Theory (ART) Networks [Gro80]. They were applied in model's identification problems but they showed great sensibility in their scale changes and orientation. Composite ANNs with great demands for their structuring, present great interest in their output's generalization in areas where the input's data are not well defined; when the appropriate methodology is found for mapping the target space data in the I/O training data (Patterns).

Bidirectional Associative Memory (BAM) Networks [Kos92]. Flexible ANNs are exploited mostly in a special type of look-up memories. Although they demand a small storage place, they convert mapping data into Patterns problems.

Brain State in a Box (BSB) Networks [A&R88]. They correlate data from a great number of inputs, by minimizing the mean-square error of a given training procedure. They perform in data/knowledge-based environments with great number of Patterns, in medical applications and in cases where it is demanded to be promoted only the one from a large amount of possible solutions.

Counterpropagation (CP) Networks [H-N88]. Successful applications range from image compression, statistical tests, observation of the stock exchange, and shares' performance rates. Their inner structure - at the end of training - resembles look-up tables.

Feed Forward (FF) Networks [A&R88]. ANNs with specific connection links between their Neurons are covered. Their adaptable capabilities and ease of implementation makes them extremely popular. The FFA-ANNs accumulate the most powerful training algorithms, the bigger R&D efforts and they tend to compose a model of comparison for most neural applications.

Hopfield Networks [Hop82]. The first ANNs that follow the evolutionary path toward the decrease of a fixed cost function. They are exploited in the memory creation, the solution of mathematical optimization problems, in simple analogue circuits (converters, amplifiers, etc.), in character recognition, and in logical problems (optimal results on travelling sales-person path).

Madaline Networks [W&L90]. They have evolved from powerfully-adjusted analogue elements that are utilized in their linear area. The simplicity and their combining capability make them capable of solving control problems, echo's cancellation in telephone systems, separation of sound signals, etc. Their adjusting structure and their accompanying Training Algorithm favours them in trade applications in the last twenty years.

Neocognitron Networks [FMI83]. Those ANNs perform smoothly when trained for identifying Chinese characters, despite their difficulties concerning varied Patterns (e.g. rotated and of different height). Even though extremely complicated in their structure, they have been a successful trade product. They can also be made to recognize Latin characters, but their use is rather limited.

Perceptron Networks [M&P69]. They are Artificial Neural Networks organized in many Slabs, reminding us of the FFA-ANN, but their Neurons are fully connected among all the Slabs. On a basis of many input Patterns, they can classify very good non-linearly separated spaces, characters, or also forms. They deal with analogue and discrete inputs but can evolve into complicated systems of higher specifications, demanding a great number of Neurons Slabs.

Self Organizing Maps (SOM) Networks [Koh84, RMS92]. Very powerful induction tools that deal with mapping patterns between differential geometric spaces. Problems of conformal mapping, through many convergence circles, result in solutions mostly unapproachable by computational means.

The ANNs that were presented above are analyzed per category in Table 1.1, where their features are also compared. Very few of them can be ANNs to be used in general applications, mostly being members of a set of specialized abilities, incapable of satisfying the full set of applications.

	Time Algorithm (C/Ds)	Design (A/D)	Architecture (F/P)	Input (F/I)	(S/nS)
ART	C/Ds	A/D	F	F/I	nS
BAM	C/Ds	A/D	P	I	S
BSB	C/Ds	D	P	I	S
CP	Ds	D	F/P	F/I	S
FFA	Ds	D	F/P	F/I	S
Hop	C/Ds	A/D	F	F/I	S
Mdl	Ds	D	P	F/I	S
Ncg	Ds	A/D	P	F/I	S
Prcp	C	A/D	F/P	F/I	S
SOM	Ds	D	P	I	nS

Adaptive Resonance Theory (ART)
Bidirectional Associative Memory (BAM)
Brain State in a Box (BSB)
Counterpropagation (CP)
Feed Forward (FFA)
Hopfield (Hop)
Madaline (Mdl)
Neocognitron (Ncg)
Perceptron (Prcp)
Self Organizing Maps (SOM)

Continuous Time: C
Discreet Time: Ds

Analogue Design: A
Digital Design: D

Full Connected Architecture: F
Partially Connected Architecture: P

Integer Input: I
Float Input: F

Supervised Training Algorithm: S
Non Supervised Training Algorithm: nS

Table 1.1: Well Known ANNs and their Characteristics

1.6 Artificial Neural Networks' Training Algorithms

Several methodologies with which the ANNs store up the discerning knowledge of a target space are provided in the bibliography. They are characterized from the specialized applications that they are developed for and from the complicated mathematical representation with regards to convergence's specifications, wanted accuracy, and integrity.

Generally, the artificial neural networks' training algorithms are not applied in a great number of different architectures; their use and structure do not permit the generalization of conclusions concerning integral rules for their use (vs. depending on the application) and do not provide any element concerning the texture of the ANN (number of Neurons/hidden Slabs, initialisation values, etc.).

The most used training algorithms follow:

Grossberg's rule [Gro80], whereby the inputs compete in order to reach the higher possible value reaching the output. This rule is characterized by the Patterns' lack in output vectors (non-supervised).

Hebbian rule [Heb49], from which the more/less contributed inputs are suitably reinforced/downgraded (correspondingly).

Hopfield's rule [Lip87], which allows the output with the higher value to direct the ANN into stability (winner takes all feature).

Kohonen's rule [Koh84], where output vectors are developed from input ones in order to satisfy a probability function. This rule too does not demand the existence of output Patterns (non supervised).

Back Propagation rule [Wer74, Par85, RHW86], whereby the wanted and real output differential error is fed back in the Weights of the previous ANN's Slabs, by using this value or its exemplar estimates of.

Widrow's rule [W&L90], which leads the ANN into a decreasing condition of the obtained mean-square output's error.

1.7 The Back Propagation Training Rule

It represents the most common training algorithm as it takes charge of the training of the widely used Perceptron and FFA-ANNs. It is usually used as the base norm for comparing the performances of neural applications. This rule [Lip87] is applied under the form of a repetitive training algorithm that tries to reduce the mean-square error of the resultant output from the wanted one. It demands a continuous Sigmoid function $\varphi(.)$, usually of the form:

$$\varphi(\zeta) = \frac{1}{1+e^{-\zeta - \Pi}}.$$ (Equation 1.3)

The algorithm is applied as follows:

Step 1   The Weights of the Synapses are set in small random values.
Step 2   The input vector $(\chi_1, \chi_2, ..., \chi_n)$ is inserted into the Network and the wanted response (output vector) $\psi_1, \psi_2, ..., \psi_m$ is enforced. Only one output (ψ_i) is usually set to the logical "1" per input vector. The I/O pairs are given to the Network individually or in sets, repeatedly.
Step 3   The actual response of the ANN is calculated (outputs $y_1, y_2, ..., y_m$).
Step 4   From the closest to the output Neurons and on, the Weights become:

$$\beta_{ij}(t+1) = \beta_{ij}(t) + \eta * \delta_j * \chi'_i.$$ (Equation 1.4)

The Weight coefficient β_{ij} links the hidden (or input) Neuron i with Neuron j, at the time instance t, the variable χ' represents either the Neuron's output or input, the coefficient η modifies the training's speed, and:

$$\delta_j = y_j * (1 - y_j) * (\psi_i - y_j) \text{ (for an output Neuron),} \qquad \text{(Equation 1.5)}$$

$$\delta_j = \chi'_j * (1 - \chi'_{ij}) * \sum_k \delta_k * \beta_{jk} \text{ (for a hidden Neuron),} \qquad \text{(Equation 1.6)}$$

where "k" indexes the Neurons situated ahead the "j" one. Usually, instead of Eq. 1.4 the more next complex type is utilized:

$$\beta_{ij}(t+1) = \beta_{ij}(t) + \eta * \delta_j * \chi'_i + \alpha * [\beta_{ij}(t) - \beta_{ij}(t-1)], 0 < \alpha < 1 \qquad \text{(Equation 1.7)}$$

"α" is chosen by the user in order to accelerate the ANN's convergence [Lip87].
Step 5   Return to step 2 for the rest of the Patterns.

1.8 The Back Propagation Rule and Kalman Filtering

The previous rule exhibits many effectiveness disadvantages during its application. Among them: **slow convergence** towards the wanted training error; **trapping** of the algorithm obtained values in local minima (as is shown in Eqns. (1.4 - 1.7) its application involves the solving of a problem of mathematical optimisation); and the **non-secure** achievement of the wanted training accuracy [Lip87], are included. Thus, its following amelioration was proposed [H&H93]:

Step 1   The biased inputs $\chi_{j-1, 0}$ of each Neuron are set in non-zero random numeric values for the Neuron's Slabs $j = 1, 2, ..., L$ and in the same amplitude the inputs are defined. Indexes "j" and "L" refer to the Neuron's Slab and the output Neuron correspondingly. Also, all the Weights in the Network are set in random initial values and a reversed table R^{-1} is initialised, usually to the unitary table I_n.
Step 2   A random input (χ_0) - output (d) Pattern of vectors are fed to the ANN.
Step 3   For the previous step Pattern the Neuron's output is calculated:

$$\psi_{jk} = \sum_{i=0}^{N} (\beta_{jki} * \chi_{j-1, i}), \qquad \text{(Equation 1.8)}$$

where $j = 1, 2, ..., L$ (Slabs of Neurons). The output of the function comes up as:

$$\chi_{jk} = \varphi(\psi_{jk}) = (1 - e^{-\alpha * \psi_{jk}}) * (1 - e^{-\alpha * \psi_{jk}}), \qquad \text{(Equation 1.9)}$$

for each Neuron "k". Index "i" (having values of 1, 2, ..., N) symbolizes the number of inputs in a Neuron, not including the biased one.

Step 4   Use of Kalman's equations. The Kalman gain is calculated first:

$$k_j = \mathbf{R}_j^{-1} * X_{j-1} * (b_j + X_{j-1}^T * \mathbf{R}_j^{-1} * X_{j-1})^{-1}, \quad \text{(Equation 1.10)}$$

for each Slab (b_j is a regulative term); table $\mathbf{R}^{-1}$ is replaced as follows:

$$[\mathbf{R}_j^{-1} - X_{j-1}^T * \mathbf{R}_j^{-1}] * b_j^{-1}. \quad \text{(Equation 1.11)}$$

Step 5 The derivative of $\varphi(\psi_{jk})$ is calculated:

$$\varphi'(\psi_{jk}) = 2 * \alpha * e^{-\alpha * \psi_{jk}} * (1 - e^{-\alpha * \psi_{jk}})^{-2}. \quad \text{(Equation 1.12)}$$

Also the following quantity (wanted and real output's difference error) is found:

$$e_{Lk} = \varphi'(\psi_{Lk}) * (d_k - \chi_{Lk}), \quad \text{(Equation 1.13)}$$

for each Neuron k. For the hidden Slabs, starting from $j = L - 1, \ldots, 1$, Eq. 1.13 is transformed in the following one:

$$e_{jk} = \varphi'(\psi_{Lk}) * [\sum_i (e_{j+1, i} * \beta_{j+1, i, k})] \quad \text{(Equation 1.14)}$$

Step 6 The following quantity is evaluated:

$$g_k = \alpha^{-1} * \ln[(1 + d_k) * (1 - d_k)^{-1}] \quad \text{(Equation 1.15)}$$

Step 7 The Weights in the Neuron's Slab output L are recalculated as follows:

$$\beta_{Lk} = \beta_{Lk} + k_L * (g_k - \psi_{Lk}) \quad \text{(Equation 1.16)}$$

For each hidden Slab the Weights are readjusted as:

$$\beta_{jk} = \beta_{jk} + k_j * e_{jk} * \mu_j. \quad \text{(Equation 1.17)}$$

where the term "μ_j" also represents a regulating training factor.

Step 8 Control of the training algorithm's effectiveness is performed by means of some criteria of convergence (distance from a norm) or also of algorithm's use for a defined number of its repetitions. In the case of the criteria's dissatisfaction or of training of all Patterns, the procedure returns to Step 2.

In comparison with the previous algorithm, this one is obviously much more complicated. The major difficulties arise from the need for the constant inversions of table $\mathbf{R}^{-1}$ and the achievement of the wanted arithmetic accuracy in the calculations. As the bibliography offers many methodologies for a table's inversion, best choice has to ultimately satisfy the application.

Experiments have shown the excellence of this algorithm when training comprised many Patterns. In those cases the convergence was successful even in a third of the previous time, often succeeding where the previous rule did not. The algorithm that used the Kalman's equations has demanded, on average, smaller Networks and has given higher accuracy. However, when used for a small number of Patterns, it proved more disadvantageous [§2.7].

1.9 Artificial Neural Networks' Application Areas
The applications of ANNs can be found in many different R&D areas. The ANNs, by excellently accomplishing classification in areas where there are not given specific rules, are applied mostly in the following R&D fields [H-N88]:
- Adapted and distributed system control for engines, artificial limbs, and of entire processes (i.e. vehicle driving, selection of starting values, etc.)
- Mathematical optimisation problems solving.
- Economical assessment and medicine for the creation of decision support systems, the modelling and the emulation of those systems.
- Image processing: transformations, compression, and storage.
- Pattern recognition (speech, characters, images, etc.), for the discovery of specific characteristics in a wide spectrum of applications.
- Synthesis and identification of natural speech.
- Data extraction (mining) from data/knowledge bases.
- Auto-, or hetero-associative memories for the structuring of storage elements that safely revoke Patterns from corrupted and/or incomplete ones.

1.10 Artificial Neural Networks in Hardware
The aforementioned ANNs architectures can be implemented both in software and in hardware environments. The reasons for an implementation choice are mostly defined so as to concur with the specifications of the particular application and will be developed extensively in the next chapters. Among them are: economical, speed of response and the promotion of the final product.

On the other hand, more developing bases arise should implementation in hardware be chosen.. As a consequence, Neural co-processors have been released that integrate one or more ANN architectures. For the same objectives, parallel processors of special purpose are also used, designs of mixed analogue/digital elements, special hardware library components (leaf cells) etc.

1.11 Artificial Neural Networks' Advantages
As the ANNs models spring from biological ones, their main qualification is focused in the way with which they store and classify Patterns and the speed with which they revoke them - an ability that results from their parallel structure. The ANNs are composed of Neurons parallel architectures so that the procedures they are applied to, inherit the advantages of parallel processing.

Most ANNs, even if they vary in Neurons, architecture, or in training algorithms, demonstrate [Koh84, Lip87, W&L90, H&H93]:

Real time training as the fed-in data are handled in times comparable to those of most processes, and can readjust their Weights accordingly.

Cross-Association of data's element they incorporate, due to their dynamic structure's storage. In that way the ANNs are capable of creating feature dependencies with which they were trained even if those features are not obvious or carefully indicated (during the ANNs' training).

Graceful degradation of the contained Patterns should some Neurons be damaged, because the ANNs converge in distributed stored data. In total, the ratio of safe-operating cases vs. damaged Neurons is large and can also be increased by the careful choice of an appropriate Network.

Generalization's abilities of Patterns' associations to whom ANNs have converged, referring into new inputs to which they are not trained. In other words, ANNs are capable of providing correct outputs by correlating unknown inputs to already-trained Patterns. This great advantage makes them ideal in applications of adjusted control and also in medical applications [E94 I-IV] [E95], as long as the choice of Patterns is done properly, so to cover "well enough" a specific region [Lip87].

Smooth operation. An ANN will converge always in its trained output-patterns if it is fed with its input-patterns, minus the training error. Moreover, it will function in the same manner and it shall always provide the closest match to its trained Patterns output, regardless of an unknown input.

Thus, based on these characteristics, the ANNs succeed to:

- Attain **real time** function during input processing. This time equals, at most, to the data's fed in one and is smaller than that of training.
- **Revoke destroyed Patterns**. ANNs achieve to converge in the correct output when input even parts of a training Pattern. Also, they can be trained by destroyed Patterns on the basis of the most important elements.
- **Recall corrupted Patterns**, while the corruption type can vary from white to random noise, in specific rates. In combination with their capability of always supplying an output, the ANNs get the better of much more demanding systems.
- Great **application speed**. Apart from its generally small training and recalling Patterns times, the whole implementation of an ANN, and the choice of the appropriate training Patterns (i.e. its incorporation in existing systems) offers more advantages than other applications. In the next chapters an analysis of comparative systems developed by the use (or not) of ANNs is offered.
- They demonstrate a very good performance in environments that are characterized by **non-linear** behaviour. ANNs solve problems of complex and complicated non-linear areas converging in the outputs, whose training Patterns indicate, based on "similar" to those taught, inputs correlations.

A comparison of ANNs vs. algorithmic applications utilization advantages, can result in the following points:

- They are shaped non-algorithmically, but can be emulated in software.
- Do not require specific rules; they "trace" them out during training.
- Integrate data storage and processing units is the same (and only) unit.
- Provide results like other powerful parallel processors.
- Adapt to eventual errors and corruptions of Patterns or structure.

- Operation is not limited by previously existent or not logical rules - their conversion into Patterns often renders novel conclusions.
- Generalize the contained elements and response into new data.
- Succeed in inner mapping (correlate) all given data (during training).
- Can satisfy many applications without significant changes in structure.
- They respond (offer an output) in a short time.

1.12 Conclusion

In this introduction, the Artificial Neural Networks are introduced. Extensive details outline the most significant of them, their capabilities, their training algorithms, and their various applications; also, the necessary terms that accompany them are given. Also provided are comparative factors of the most known of them, their differences, and in the application area for each of them.

The clarification of ANN's role, the need for their utilization, and furthermore the mathematical analysis of the equations that describe their function is not the purpose of this Chapter. More interesting was the hinting to their usefulness in practical applications, the importance of the solutions they offer, and the multi-dimensional perception of the application's space they offer. The extensive bibliography that co-exists covers the needs of the interested reader.

1.13 References

[McC43]   McCulloch, W. S. and Pitts, W., "A Logical Calculus of the Ideas Immanent in Nervous Activity", Bull. of Math. Bioph., vol. 5, pp. 115-133, 1943.
[Heb49]   Hebb, D. O., The Organization of Behavior, Wiley, New York, 1949.
[M&P69]   Minsky, M. and Papert, S., Perceptrons, MIT Press, Cambridge, 1969.
[Wer74]   Werbos, P. J., Beyond Regression: New Tools for Prediction and Analysis in the Behavioral Sciences, Ph.D. Thesis, Harvard University, Cambridge, 1974.
[Gro80]   Grossberg, S., "How Does a Brain Build a Cognitive Code?", Psychol. Rev., vol. 87, pp. 1-51, 1980.
[Hop82]   Hopfield, J. J., "Neural Networks and Physical Systems with Emergent Collective Computational Abilities", Proc. Nat. Acad. of Sciences, vol. 79, pp. 2554-2558, 1982.
[FMI83]   Fukushima, K., Miyake, S., and Ito, T., "Neocognitron: A Neural Network Model for a Mechanism of Visual Pattern Recognition", IEEE Trans. on SMC, vol. 13, pp. 826-834, 1983.
[Koh84]   Kohonen, T., Self-Organization and Associative Memory, Springer-Verlag, Berlin, 1984.
[Par85]   Parker, D., Learning Logic, TR-87, MIT Press, Cambridge, 1985.
[RHW86]   Rumelhart, D. E., Hinton, G. E., and Williams R. J., "Learning Internal Representations by Error Propagation", Parallel Distributed Processing: Explorations in the Microstructure of Cognition, vol. 1, pp. 318-362, MIT Press, Cambridge, 1986.
[Lip87]   Lippmann, R. P., "An Introduction to Computing with NN", IEEE ASSP Magazine, vol. 5, pp. 4-22, 1987.

[A&R88]	Anderson, J. A. and Rosenfeld, E., (editors), Neurocomputing: Foundations of Research, MIT Press, Cambridge, 1988.
[H-N88]	Hecht - Nielsen, R., "Neurocomputing: Picking the Human Brain", IEEE Spectrum, vol. 25(3), pp. 36-41, 1988.
[Vem88]	Vemuri, V., (editor), Artificial Neural Networks: Theoretical Concepts, IEEE Computer Society Press, 1988.
[Pao89]	Pao, Y.-H., Adaptive Pattern Recognition and Neural Networks, Addison-Wesley, Reading, 1989.
[W&L90]	Widrow, B. and Lehr, M. A., "30 years of Adaptive NN: Perceptron, Madaline, and Backpropagation", Proc. of the IEEE, vol. 23, pp. 1415-1442, 1990.
[F&S91]	Freeman, J. A. and Skapura, D. M., Neural Networks: Algorithms, Applications, and Programming Techniques, Addison-Wesley, Reading, 1991.
[Kos92]	Kosko, B., Neural Networks for Signal Processing, Prentice-Hall, New Jersey, 1992.
[RMS92]	Ritter, H., Martinetz, T., and Schulten, K., Neural Computation and Self-Organizing Maps, Addison-Wesley, Reading, 1992.
[H&H93]	Hush, D. R. and Horne, B. G., "Progress in Supervised NN", IEEE Sig. Proc. Mag., vol. 10, pp. 8-39, 1993.
[E94 I]	Economou, G. - P. K., Spiropoulos, K., Economopoulos, N. M., Charokopos, N., Lymberopoulos, D., Spiliopoulou, M., Haralambopulu, E., and Goutis, C. E., "Medical Diagnosis and Artificial Neural Networks: A Medical Expert System applied to Pulmonary Diseases", Proc. of 1994 IEEE Int. Work. on NNSP, pp. 482 - 489, Ermioni, Greece, Sep. 1994.
[E94 II]	Economou, G. - P. K., Spiropoulos, K., Economopoulos, N. M., Charokopos, N., Lymberopoulos, D., Spiliopoulou, M., Haralambopulu, E., and Goutis, C. E., "Medical Decision Making Systems in Pulmonology: A Creative Environment based on Artificial Neural Networks", Proc. of 1994 IEEE Int. Conf. on SMC, pp. 975 - 980, San Antonio, USA, Oct. 1994.
[E94 III]	Economou, G. - P. K., Spiropoulos, K., Economopoulos, N. M., Charokopos, N., Zikos, P., Lymberopoulos, D., and Goutis, C. E., "Decision Supporting Systems in Medical Diseases' Diagnosis: An Artificial Neural Networks Approach", Proc. of Annual Fall Meeting of the Biomedical Society, pp. 123 - 129, Tempe, USA, Oct. 1994.
[E94 IV]	Economou, G. - P. K., Economopoulos, N. M., Charokopos, N., Zikos, P., Lymberopoulos, D., Spiropoulos, K., and Goutis, C. E., "Suggesting Diagnosis of Diseases and Treatment: How far Artificial Neural Networks can go?", Proc. of 1994 IEEE ISANN, pp. 626 - 631, Tainan, Taiwan, Dec. 1994.
[E95]	Economou, G. - P. K., Economopoulos, N. M., Lymberopoulos, D., and C. E. Goutis, "Experiences Accumulated Working towards Medical Decision Support Systems", J. of Microprocessing and Microprogramming, vol. 40, pp. 883-886, 1995.

2nd Chapter

Decision Support Systems

Man is the last continent…
Ed Cooper

2.1 Introduction

Decision support systems (DSSs) have flourished greatly during the last decade in the fields of R&D spanning many areas of science, technology, and health, mostly because of the need to attain "good enough" choices within a limited time [J&F90]. Those Systems are developed wherever there is need for decision making depending on a large number of complicated elements that the human mind usually succeeds with more than satisfying results [B&C83].

Our search for the representation of human experience/expertise and the simulation of logical feature's extraction from DSSs has resulted in an original system that is based on a combination of FFA-ANNs. It possesses qualities that permit its application in whichever selected field of human experience that is characterized by organised structures. The architecture of this system follows a modular structure. In that way, it provides an appropriate environment for the study of other different systems, mapping their behaviour by means of appropriate interfaces that are related with each application.

2.2 Necessity for Structuring Decision Support Systems

The extensive concentration of R&D towards the utilization of those Systems coincides essentially with the extended use of personal computers as the necessary tools for a researcher. Through them, the resultant cost of an application decreases so such that the request for better control in process analysis and survey are promoted more systematically and in larger scale.

In specialised as well as in more general technology's sectors, experienced users need decision support systems [Mar88] for the tracking and **exploration** of systems' response that appear to be complicated and dependent on a great number of different parameters. In that case, decision support systems become the **experiment bases** for the improvement of systems' function and performance conditions and the adjustment of parameters that would not be possible to be altered as a part of the applications they affect.

Therefore, the Systems offer the expert an autonomous environment when **simulating control rules** of running processes could not be made to cease their operation for study reasons. From the application simulations of those processes by means of DSS, the processing of **large application data** can be achieved, whose importance and function's process special role are unknown. On the other hand, off-line simulations decrease the demand for a great deal of processing time. Finally, the use of DSS provides **safe** simulation conditions and exploiting of evolutionary rules starting from application models.

At the same time, DSSs were developed [Mar88] for the analysis of "rules of thumb" as they evolve from human experience in the application fields. DSSs can be found at the base of diagnostic systems but they are also applied so that **products of induction** can be standardised (in their description, analysis, and simulation). Since DSSs are real-time systems, they directly interfere with an application, in order to recommend the proper evolution process in the implementation field, and demonstrate great induction abilities.

DSSs are founded on the basis of specific-purpose computational devices or by using low-cost material. Being structural at the core, they can generalize already known Patterns into unknown inputs, using their ability to operate as comparators-controllers of applications that have similarities with the ones that (the Systems) are already trained to.

Furthermore, their planning specifications tend to ensure the researcher-designer, as well as the specialist and the end user, coverage of a number of parameters as far as application enrichment is concerned. The function of decision induction, that simulates the expert's one, is a differential factor to conventional programming and constitutes a must-fulfilled need.

The input data are fed to a System and are symbolically processed, as they are "translated" into an inner (**symbolic**) mapping of, and inside, the DSS [K&P89]. Conventional programming comprises of syntax and application structures that do not ascribe to the induction application in a satisfactory manner.

The **pre-processing of application data** is another training parameter; data are usually a subject of re-arrangements [§2.3] in order to be utterly exploited. This procedure is facilitated by the use of Systems because they support structures that are equivalent to the elements' traits [K&P89].

The most important requirement concerning the Systems, as expressed by experts, is not related on their accuracy as much as in the full covering of the application domain. A System's **flexibility**, as a parameter, associates its training by Patterns that the expert certificates are sufficient, as well as the confrontation of competitive cases in order for a DSS to always respond.

Conversely, the **expansibility** of a System is an important factor right from its implementation. Modern developing perception **anticipates** the creation of Systems that, through some changes, will be capable to cope with different applications. The system structure should anticipate further developing skills.

Moreover, a decision support system should periodically readjust to new facets of the environment it is attuned. Thus, it should exhibit **multifaceted learning capabilities**, working methodologies that cover a certain domain, and detract probable contradictory rules (or features), redundancy of structure, and un-correspondent rules following the required response achievement.

A System's **access** into model databases for their eventual completion is also sought, as well as uncomplicated **interfacing** with this access (between expert-System -friendly user interface, System-database, etc.). In addition, a System should have the means to accomplish **portability** in other computing environments or application areas, quick **mapping** to different hardware structures, and conformity to working specifications in environments where **adverse operating conditions** are dominating (due to temperature, dust, noise, etc.).

2.3 Decision Support Systems' Basic Structures

The first stage in the development of those Systems is the **extraction** of experts' experience. Then follow its **representation, mapping**, and **pre-processing** stages in order to form training Patterns. The second stage usually refers to the transformation of often vague data, always provided by the expert, in clear reference domains and the fourth to arranging these elements (i.e. images' regions of interest, normalization of values, etc.) so that some of their components can be highlighted. The third stage has already been defined - training of a DSS [§1.3]. The above scheme is completed by providing an interface environment that will undertake the data exchange between the specialist, the user, and the System, through the choice of a proper form and layout.

Even between specialists of the same field, many arguments arise about the number and the nature of parameters, their definition, their importance, and the form of their representation, the accuracy by which they are expressed, and the questioning of their use. Also, the shortage of specific reference models leads to expertise data standardization that is not widely acceptable.

Decision support systems can be developed in general purpose software and hardware environments, by means of more or less specialized structures or a platform that serves other Systems. There are exploited as parts of control, classification, standardization systems, etc. [W&K84], through the use of many implementation, simulation, and induction techniques.

DSSs are made up from several sub-systems, the **knowledge base** that incorporates the data of fields the Systems are mapped; the **inference engine** that exploits the knowledge base by means of rules; specialized sections that assume **data exchange** between the "outer world", the user, and the researcher. Fig. 2.1 presents the general structure of a decision support system.

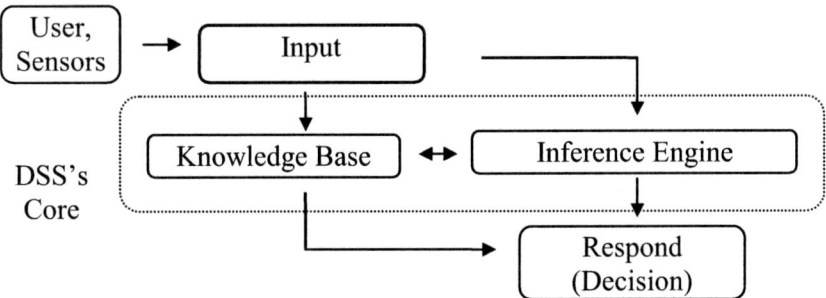

Figure 2.1: Decision Support System - General Structure

The System's data exchange with its "outer world" (environment), the experts, the users, and the researchers, is a topic of a special technology branch - the interface development between human beings and devices. Beyond the friendliness it must present, it should ensure some abilities to justify the final response (decision) and analysis of its output (induced) route.

Based on the above, **communication protocols** between elements of the System's core, the inputs, the decisions, and the researchers are developed. They correlate statistical data, database information, etc. or they refer to technical elements.

Reference models are also developed that provide standardization of the characterization of sub-sets' processing, of the development steps, and of the System's operation. However, often, those steps are skipped and a system is structured without proper standardization. This lack of standards deters the collaborating efforts between different specialists' teams [K&P89, E93 III].

Finally, **single user environments** (graphical, etc.) are developed. Those are ensued from different experts' and users' ergonomic fashions in their respective work fields, as well as from the enhancement of their knowledge.

The system development researcher has the key-role for the creation of a decision support system. The expertise's representation, the DSS's implementation, and input's feeding comprise his/her application domain, and the System should not be altered without his/her supervision. Fig. 2.2 sums up the interaction between end users, Systems, experts, and researchers.

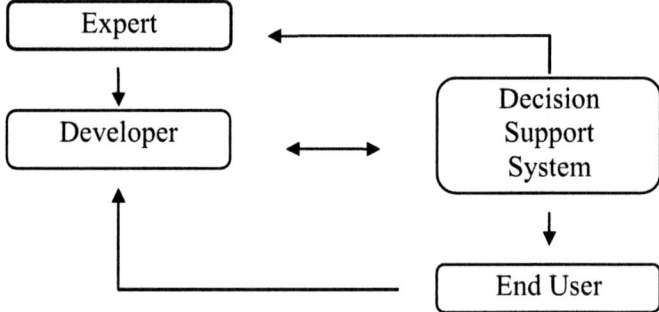

Figure 2.2: Interaction during DSSs' Structuring

2.4 Decision Support Systems' Training

The induction ability of these Systems is designed in order to cover a wide spectrum of new cases and to "reach a decision" by means of processing their knowledge base through controlling its techniques. For this purpose, they contain data that come from an application, pre-processed or not, as well as (other) elements from the system development researcher or the expert knowledge that are not necessarily related with the application [Mar88]. The latter are probable to encumber the System's ability to respond, its portability, etc. Moreover, the collaboration between researchers and experts is effectively promoted since they agree in a common terminology and practice.

From a system's point of view, related to a researcher, a System processes the protogenic-provided experience (of an expert) and converts it into an inner mapping in its knowledge base, by use of: **symbols** (with explicit report and characteristics of everyday practice), **linguistic rules**, and association and handling **syntax** of these elements (symbols rules).

The System ensures the inner account of expertise by means of rules that use, standardize, and interpret symbols and thus represent the application field concepts. This is succeeded by means of **logic rules** (prepositional, disjunction, and categorical reasoning), **structured knowledge representation** (semantic networks, frames, conceptional dependence, and description of successive facts) and knowledge of **procedural representation** [K&P89].

A DSS induces decisions as the inference engine handles the knowledge base by exploiting its symbolic build up. The DSS responds by means of reasoning structures that are **non-cumulative** (not reviewing previous rules), non-certain (scalable/fuzzy, probabilistic, and entropic in nature), and **heuristic**, that are overall referred to as **control techniques** (of a knowledge base) [K&P89]. Those techniques structure the base in search graphs or trees.

From the standpoint of experience *per se* - in the way that the expert provides it - a decision support system is organized based on the principle of the reproduction of its inferential work out. Different techniques that have dissimilar reasoning (structure of experience) as well as ways to accomplish the extraction of the decision, apply as stated by the circumstance [K&P89].

As mentioned before, seeking the experience that has been stored in a knowledge base is actualised by means of control techniques. Their utilization solves a specific problem that would demand huge portions of time should the whole area the knowledge base is to cover, was to be explored. If the bases are to be structured in tree forms, the most extensive used methods are [K&P89]:

- By **depth first**. Starting from an initial condition, the structuring moves on in order to cover a whole branch of the tree before it regresses.
- By **breadth first**. The research exhausts all the branches of the tree that are placed at the same level of importance, before it continues.
- By **best node first**. By means of specific criteria, an initiative branch is chosen; from it the rest of the tree springs, depending on the criteria.
- By **partial constraint satisfaction**. Based on this, any control technique is exploited to shape the tree whether some partial restrictions are first satisfied.
- By **means-ends analysis**. On the basis of numeric criteria, the shortest distance between following and previous branches of the tree is chosen.
- By **min-max algorithms**. They are applied mostly to game theory and are trying to assess competing rules in order to expand the tree.
- By **bandwidth first**. Its application is focused on the lessening of a distance (width) from the final decision in order to decrease the research time.
- By **nearest neighbour first**. During the research, the finding of the best following branch within the neighbour of the previous branch is tracked down.
- By **branching and bounding** the route that leads to the decision (intermediate or final), so that the best (or even provisional) path between the already tested branches with a new one is continuously compared.

To recapitulate, decision support systems offer a human experience (specialized knowledge) mapping in a form that automatically reproduces it and fairly resembles the biological induction. They have an advantage concerning the **handling of application data**, since conventional programming does not offer the same mapping, detection, and specification capabilities.

Furthermore, the **correlation** of all the elements that compose the knowledge base usually represents the basis where the choice of a System's application is relayed. DSSs can demonstrate the user the way their decision was reached by recording the "path" that has led to it, offering backing-up services.

2.5 Decision Support Systems' Disadvantages

A system's researcher/developer has to carefully research requirements such as Systems supplies, before he/she favours a selection. Disadvantages from DSSs' use can also turn up as the shortage of some parameter's standardization is not uncommon and depends on the application [Alt87].

Systems that are developed with regards to the principles of Section 2.4 usually result in large sizes of their knowledge base, especially when specialized methods for the reinforcement of the System's effectiveness are used (e.g. normalizations). As a consequence, the System's implementation is complicated. Moreover, the non-standardized mapping and representation of data fed makes the linking to similar Systems range from difficult at best. The developing techniques, for better response reasons, use to take profit of the individuality traits of a computational environment vs. the implementation generality, depriving the System of maintenance and further R&D facilities.

The clarity in the backing-up of the "logical" cohesion that leads to a System's decision, that is one of the most important advantages of DSSs, can constitute a non-usable characteristic. The way to construct rules and control techniques is non-standard even among researchers and does not permit extended conclusions justification on the performance of DSSs, due to their specialized (symbolic) structure. Thus, the existence of a common model describing language (that does not exist) seems necessary. Besides, when expertise is mapped on those rules, some alterations to the actual application's handling are inserted too as the researcher's and the expert's aspects are also introduced into the data.

The standardization of the intermediate decisions are also reached by the inference engine, which tends to make a System inflexible when the application's peculiarities are not considered. Most Systems tend to remain adherent to their corresponding fields, exploiting special features, making their generalization into other fields time-consuming, tiring, and dubious. The inference engine itself follows a logic of supplying a response which, when achieved, cuts off any other effort (as the specialist's experience would have already been applied). Further System operation usually assumes the collaboration between different teams of experts, a factor that adds to the System implementation time and is hindered by the lack of application data standardization.

In this sense, these traditional Systems inhibit direct data exchange, a routine characterizing the experts during their collaboration. Even the creation of many similar Systems for the same application, being based on different specialists so that DSSs could complement each other, does not come close to such a qualification. An implementation would not have the means to provide for the comparison of variations or (possible) new cases, and would create partial decision dominance or problems in evaluation parameters.

Additionally, experts in order to give their opinions on a problem, usually employ a draft reference model. Consequently, for a more thorough evaluation of elements and support of their decision, they take advantage of the application of more standardised rules. This methodology cannot be put into traditional DSSs as their integration demands a great deal of application knowledge that is usually not available (or not standardised).

Conversely, the utilization of these draft reference models by a System would complicate the effort for the generalization of a specific architecture even more. Being strictly specialized models, they are applied in other fields, mostly as a base of inductance comprehension and not as a rule.

Because of their structure, the decision support systems develop their inference engine by means of control techniques that elaborate the knowledge base by means of its rule cohesion. On the other hand, the techniques' choices qualify, depending on the rules priority in the case of an inconsistency. This operation is barely based on the evaluation of the whole expert's knowledge tree; on the other hand, the expert is probably not interested in the complete coverage of the application field. Thus, this approach includes the danger of an unstable System or a counterproductive operation of the System in the long run.

In addition, time, as a capital variable, usually is not adequately dealt with. Decisions that have been made on the way towards the final ones, are barely reviewed before a System "re-reads" its input. Moreover, applications and Systems change as time elapses, being unable to respond to the same characteristics or with the same effectiveness, so demanding frequent upgrading of their knowledge base to ensure a smooth operation. A DSS's adaptability to these changes is not easily attained because of the nature of the rules that are set *a priori*.

Finally, Systems' adaptability in cases that are not anticipated and also their generalization into other fields, are some additional subjects concerning the systems' researchers. The nature of the human abilities' functions of correlation, induction, and elements' cross-checking that lead to a decision even with the use of unknown data, by the core and the qualities of well known applications, is not achieved by means of traditional DSSs [Alt87].

2.6 The Contribution of Artificial Neural Networks

The recent utilization of ANNs on a large scale, shows their credentials and great appropriateness to further develop the most promising applications of **artificial intelligence techniques**: the decision support and also more general systems [Hil90]. Their training, through examples of input and output pairs (Patterns), play to their advantage; the characteristics that have already been mentioned [§1.11] compose a remarkable implementation base.

In this book, a methodology is presented for the development of DSSs that are based on ANNs. Research in this area was preferred because of these Networks' qualities as well as in an effort to wipe out some Systems disadvantages, as previously stated [§2.5].

As the base of the proposed new System, the FFA-ANN was been preferred; FFA-ANN is very easily implemented because of its **partial serial structure**.

This means that some of its Neurons practically do not need to operate at the same time, i.e. they can be alternated. Correspondingly, during the hardware implementation of FFA-ANNs, chip space reduction is accomplished due to the fact that the implementing ANNs' connections are exclusively related to the actual functioning Neurons, without reducing its effectiveness [§6.5].

Also, the training algorithms for FFA-ANNs are being continually under further development. As a conclusion, faster, more accurate, and more easily implemented software and hardware techniques are presented from many researchers [§4.4|6|8, §5.8]. Usually they exploit unique application qualities, such as the cohesion of final output ranking and not the accuracy of that ranking [§6.4].

Due to the FFA-ANN's structure, its training algorithms are implemented very productively in **different hardware and software environments** [§1.7|8, §6.5]. Conclusively, the software on which it is simulated presents adaptation qualities when transferred from computer to computer (PC-MSDOS, HP/Apollo-HPUX and HP/Apollo-Domain_OS) and as far as the hardware issue is concerned, there is no demand for use of special elements. Despite all of these drawbacks, the architectural simplicity that characterizes the Network [§6.6] allows the use of special purpose sub-programs/circuits with better performances related to the implementation convenience, speed, and output accuracy.

FFA-ANNs ensure many of the wanted qualities of decision support systems as they induce conclusions concerning their training and new inputs [Hil90]. Furthermore, they also integrate in their structure:

Operations in parallel. ANNs that consist of a partial serial structure in the transmission of their data from Slab to Slab [§1.2], e.g. the FFA-ANN elaborate their inputs in parallel (i.e. among Neurons of the same Slab).

Dynamic storage of elements. Experience is accumulated in FFA-ANNs in the Weights of their Synapses. It is classified and accessed with the convergence of input data vs. the Patterns by which they were trained.

Robustness. The distribution in its Weights' values training Patterns contributes towards the proper function of an FFA-ANN, within adjustable limits, even after the destruction of an important part of the Network in a random manner.

Generalization abilities into new inputs. FFA-ANNs provide high reliability in responses after being fed inputs to which they were not trained.

Very good response times. Training periods are always time-demanding but of smaller duration than other artificial intelligence techniques.

Even greater **tolerance** in mistaken, fuzzy, and inaccurate inputs than other Systems, that varies according to the type of failure.

In contrast, traditional Systems tend to not present the above qualities in the same degree. Bibliography shows they perform only where the application is well defined [Hil90]. The use of FFA-ANNs negates the problem, given that a capable number of training Patterns is provided, and the Systems based on them reach convergence within a short time [Hil90, E94 II]. Finally, although Systems are exploited in a very "narrow" environment, the FFA-ANN is easily and widely used in other applications and has a more "open" structure [Hay94].

Hence, this book was focused on the creation of a decision support system of general application that would be based on FFA-ANNs. That System is presented in the next chapters thoroughly and exploits, in the best way, the advantages of both referential fields of artificial intelligence techniques: the classic expert system and the artificial neural networks.

2.7 The Basic Artificial Neural Network

A large number of ANNs [Lip87] have been simulated using C programming language - towards finding the best Network candidate which would compose the basic System's ANN. **Experimental data** prejudged the FFA-ANN, with three (3) total Slabs, based on the features it demonstrated during **training**, **expansion** of its inputs and Synapses, and the **convergence speed** of its Weights to the chosen I/O Patterns.

Two classic algorithms have been chosen to readjust the Weights of FFA-ANNs: the back propagation rule [Lip87] and the application of Kalman's equations to the above with some improvements (mostly in initialisation issues) [S&T92]. The two algorithms were presented and studied widely in Chapter 1 [§1.7|8], where a comparison is been made of their advantages.

The algorithm that included the Kalman's equations dominated the experiments [E94 I-II], [E95] in **initialisation handiness** of training parameters and **smooth behaviour** during the rule's application. Changes were not needed in the Patterns' series, nor a special random selection for the Weights' initial values and important interference in the back propagation classic rule parameters - necessary elements for the convergence of this rule.

Furthermore, the back propagation rule failed to achieve **convergence** for all the experiments, mostly because of the vast number of Patterns that characterized the application. This number of Patterns was decided necessary by the experts' team so that the whole application area could be covered. These Patterns were derived from doctors' experience and also from medical elements of patients at the General Regional University Hospital of Patras [§3.8.1]. Differences occurred in handling training Patterns as well. The first algorithm cannot readjust the FFA-ANN Weights fed with many pairs of training Patterns.

Concerning the training speed, the second algorithm takes over again the first only when the **Patterns** have many components. In the opposite case, the "simple" back propagation training rule prevails. This happens because the adjusting Kalman's equations (filtering back propagation ones) demand some function circles before they begin to converge towards the final value.

Finally, the aforementioned training techniques varied in **convergence accuracy**, too. Most of the times, the second algorithm succeeded to achieve convergence with a lower final training error and same amount of time.

2.8 Requirements for a Novel Decision Support System

The specifications that were set for the conception, creation, and implementation of a new Decision support system were more related to the importance of the experience itself. The goal was to manage its use in the application fields that it was trained for, in order to continue to develop and evolve.

General modulation principles for mapping expertise in ANNs' training Patterns are given, based on choices that tend towards standardization [E95].

Human experience is based on a primary theoretical knowledge around the functioning, practice, or also the special field characteristics to which it is referring. This theoretical knowledge comes from the training that is received in the field where the human being develops, and is completed in the working environment. It comprises the **model** on which the decision will be based.

This model is composed of features such as the **application structures**. It concerns the flow of a decision and the data that lead to, classify, and describe it due to intra-correlation. Data's exploitation is an important System developing factor, having to support the application structures.

The model is tested in working conditions thanks to the attrition with whichever problems arise. These are usually characterized by the unexpected event of a new demand and the expert is called to induce some new confrontation rules based on the criteria of his experience to date. His obligation is to extract a solution in a predefined (short) time. This demand, if combined with the rest application needs, hinders a System structuring. These steps comprise the stage of **adaptation** which controls experience.

New data are being processed from the more general to the more specific, composing the **new model**. Also, the System evolves, adjusts, and develops constantly, according to application demands. Usually it is reduced to specialized bonds, always directing its function towards the reach of a solution.

On the other hand, usually the application of human experience follows the utilization of some criteria, more or less standard. "Rules of thumb" help human beings in memorizing a series of rules, although they detract his cogitative ability as time passes by. Thus, a particular rule is not recalled, but rather the conditions it was first introduced to, along with its implicit results.

Consequently, a series of additional qualities that should characterize the new DSS appear. The first refers to its structure – this is why the **modular** [Hay94]. Modules' development paybacks in less training speed, when the application field can be broken into sub-sets (structures). Each separate module is separated into that sub-set and ignores whatever does not refer to that. Even if the application has complicated structures, a modular system approach can provide the appropriate analysis field, so that new elements can appear. Also, mapping the experience into training Patterns is less difficult (whatever is in excess is ignored, whereas the specific is highlighted). Such a modular topology simulates the brain's physiology [Hay94].

The System's **adaptability** in different application fields is an important factor for its evaluation. Decision support systems are not developed in such general structures so as to fit many (different) fields requirements, since they do not preserve their effectiveness, but they own to expand their inputs and to applications that are characterized by similar structures. Modularity permits such a feature as it simplifies the System's structure [Hay94].

Another demanded System's characteristic consists of its ability to provide the end users with the series of **"logical speculations"** that directs it to respond with a specific set of sub- to final decision. Thus, decisions "backing-up" is crucial.

The intermediate steps should demonstrate the System's induction function with clarity, completeness, and through reference models. At the same time and during the process of new inputs by the System, the expert should be able to interfere and discriminate some of these elements - erasing the effect of others.

2.9 The Novel Decision Support System

The new DSS, shown in Fig. 2.3, permits the assignment of structured operations to its processing hierarchy strata (Layers, Levels, Slabs), as ensued from the application's organization. It is fed by a specialist's experience that it allocates throughout its processing chain of command (Fig. 2.3, "ellipses", "circles"). The connections between these levels depend on and are defined from the application, and only the first ones accept the **offered input** to the System, which is **partially** allocated to them, depending on their importance. Other processing layers can be "tuned" to respond with **selected intermediate outputs** that will doubtless generate likewise consistent **inputs** throughout the next layers.

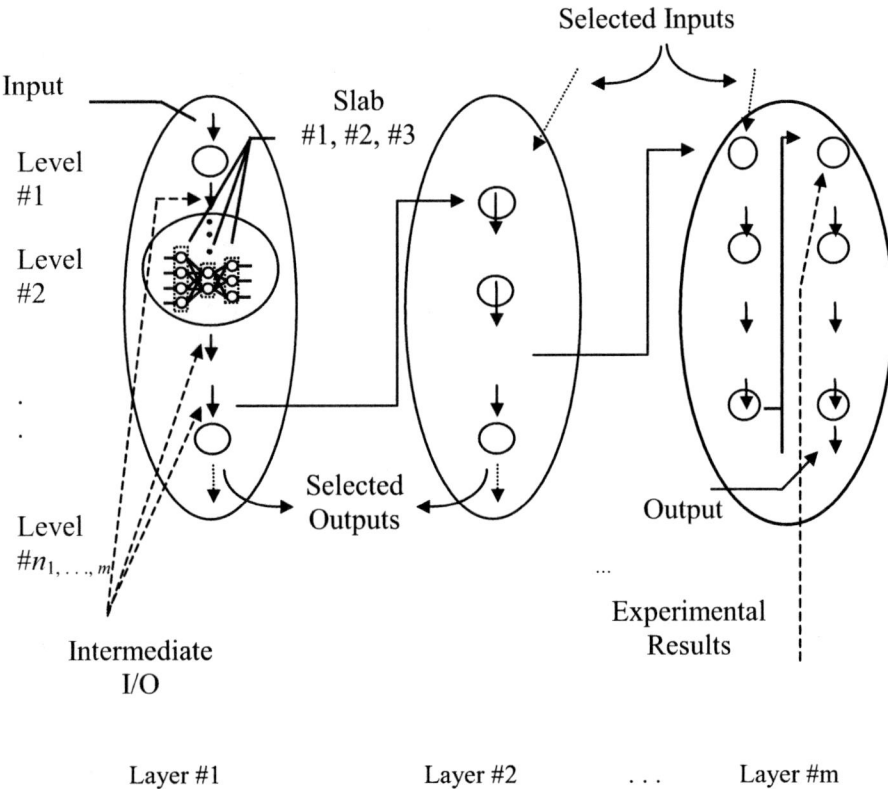

Figure 2.3: The Novel Decision Support System

The novel DSS is made of hierarchical strata, the **Layers** (Fig. 2.3, "ellipses"), equal in number to the application group of outputs from the more general to more specific structures. A final Layer at the end of the chain compares the experiment, test (in case of a medicine field), or control data of any sort of results that are requested for the support and confirmation of a decision of a Layer (Fig. 2.3, double series of "circles"). During this comparison, the Layer that has edited the pre-final decision (indexed as "$m - 1$") is enriched with the experimental results that are inserted in separate series of ANNs' levels in the final Layer; its "normal" and "enriched" outputs are then aggregated.

By this, the System adapts and takes care of time and experimental results. At the same time, the clarity in intermediate and final decisions extraction is dominant, due to the modularity of the System's structure that permits the observation of its operation output per output.

Each Layer is organized in hierarchical sub-strata, the **Levels** (Fig. 2.3, "circles"). These are implemented through series of FFA-ANNs (the modules of the novel System), that accept inputs and intermediate decisions and respond according to their specialization. The Levels' outputs vary from specifying subsets to constitute sub-decisions and (partial) actions.

The System Networks' connections (from Slab to Slab) and training are defined in relation to the application field. The feeding to the System of the appropriate training Patterns must face possible problems, such as the shortage of unambiguous rules/examples, of standardized element data, and of the degrading of input data quality within the different process levels [E95].

The System route towards the extraction of the final decision is represented by means of the Networks' outputs in such a manner that it turns up clear, ready to train a specialized user, be confirmed by an expert one, etc. The expert can intervene in the way that the elements lead to the decisions within a stratum and favour some outputs than others, depending on his/her expertise. Despite this option, an expert should not be let to train a System alone [§4.4|6|8].

The utilization of this specified architecture, guarantees the decision support system's **adaptability** in new, different application fields because of its structure that follows the application organization's ones and the use of FFA-ANNs. Virtually, finding the appropriate training Patterns represents the only important problem. Employment of series of modules (FFA-ANNs) that "weigh" intermediate decisions leads towards the final one's induction, decreases the connections, and offer an architecture that is adjusted to different applications.

Moreover, this architecture offers **speed** in decision's induction concerning new inputs. The experiments that have been conducted have shown that when connection multiplicity and the number of Neurons and Synapses increase, speed decreases by a smaller ratio than that corresponding to the traditional Systems during the augmentation of their knowledge base.

The System's **generalization** into new training Patterns and applications, since Networks can be repeatedly trained, conveys yet another advantage.

As it will later shown [§6.11], by simply setting the appropriate Weights in a specific System of a similar topology (that has already been implemented in hardware), the System can be adjusted to cover the requirements that different applications "command" (i.e. retargeting). It covers connections between ANNs' Neurons, ANNs to ANNs, evaluation issues, etc.

The novel System is totally **transparent** in its route to favour the appropriate output Pattern (taught or induced one). As the hierarchy of input data processing has been anticipated, this route's utilization is made in each stratum separately, either in Layers, or in Levels, or in FFA-ANNs.

On the other hand, the excessive amount in processing modules (ANNs) that are present remain the main disadvantage of this DSS. Yet, it can be ultimately shown that this **would not** amount to a prohibited evolution factor as software/hardware arrangements can seriously limit their number [§3.8|9, §6.5].

2.10 Comparison with the Adaptive Expert Network

The bibliography offer verys few examples of combined artificial neural networks and decision support systems. ANNs and DSSs are separately treated and only highlighted are the advantages for each being chosen in specific applications, allaying their single disadvantages according to the implementation area. Analyses can also be found for their unattached use, considering ANNs apart from the rest of artificial intelligence techniques [B&C83]. The reasons are detected in the structure and the up-to-date applications of Systems and Networks.

Then again, Haykin [Hay94] also proposed a modular structure of a system of **adaptive expert networks** that are based on ANNs and gating networks ("weighting" partial results), and simple accumulators [Fig. 2.4]. Each of those networks (ANNs and gating ones), are trained in order to implement a special correlation of their inputs and outputs, so that the next gating networks would permit the dispatching of ANN's outputs or the intermediate accumulators, forwards in the system's hierarchy structuring.

The difference between Haykin's system application and the one presented in this book mainly lies in the way all these networks (inter)connect. Each of the ANNs and the gating networks of Haykin's, **is fed all the input vectors** during the training and the use of the system. Later on, the ANNs that are situated in the first processing stages, are chosen to become sensitive in some input constituents (through the training process). The gating networks are consequently chosen to weight (through properly selected individual or non- coefficients) the total ANNs' outputs, depending on the scale of the fed input data. The gating networks' outputs are weighted from the next gating networks, until the final stages of the system and the application demands are completed [Hay94].

The novel System presented in this book introduces hierarchy constructs in the input process from the start (as defined by the expert) and allocates the ANNs' specialization by partially defining inputs to each of them. The "weighting" and the calculation of intermediate decisions are made from the next artificial neural networks - identical in structure and in abilities with the previous ones. Any ANN could be the base ANN, not a specific one as in the adaptive expert network, further inconsistent to the gating network [Hay94].

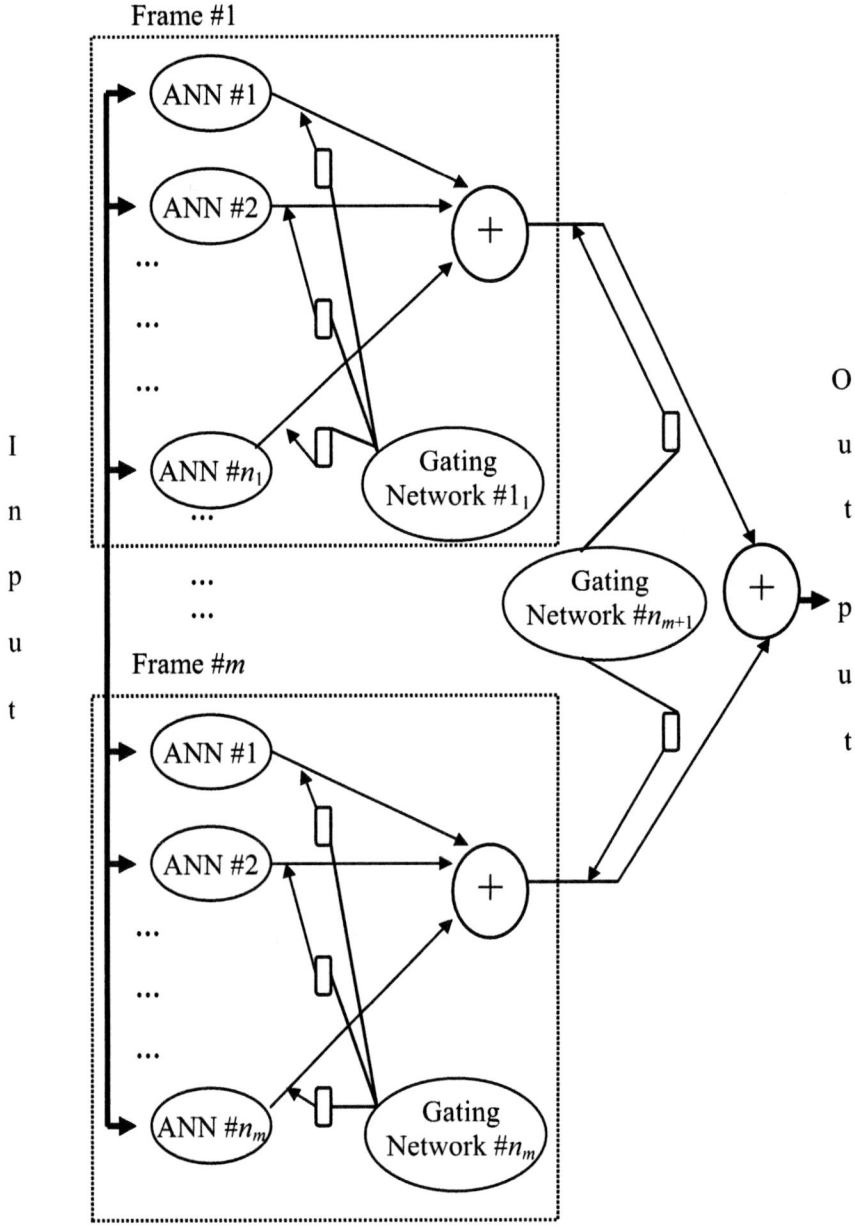

Figure 2.4: A Section of Haykin's Adaptive Expert Network

Furthermore, Haykin tries to prove the inductive force of ANNs with no hidden Slabs - a DSS based on modules composed of only one (1) Neuron Slab. According to the R&D experts on artificial neural networks [Lip87, A&R88, Hil90, Kos92, S&T92], their ability to generalize and to correlate data fed through I/O Patterns lies to a great extent in their hidden Slab. Therefore, the Haykin's approach only flourishes where the modelling of an area is completely known *a priori* and the suggestion of non-evident rules is not demanded, so that the appropriate association for the gating networks and the training models is well defined.

Such a decision support system's architecture cannot be generalized into other applications after being mapped to an individual one (too much peculiarities have been already handled), and remains bounded to its explicit needs. On the contrary, as it will be shown in the next sessions, this book's novel System is equipped with a suitable structure that permits its adaptation to other applications where the parameters of a new area problem are similar to the existing inputs, outputs and the ANNs that create the strata of another area's data [§3.8|9, §6.11]. As already mentioned, the System shall adapt to the new area's requirements as soon as the training Patterns and methodology will be made available.

2.11 Conclusion

The presentation of a novel decision support system is the first contribution of this book. Research results on artificial neural networks traits' comparison were focused more towards a higher, abstract development level than solely ANNs' links: the finding of the appropriate structures and their connections in order to compose the architecture of a proper system. This method was considered compulsory as the ANNs are examined as completed tools for an application's development. Their abilities permit the generalization and representation of the structures of an application, as it is given in the next chapter.

The presented System has been based on a specific architecture, the FFA-ANN, after research for a better profitability between different network topologies [§2.6]. The same has happened with the Networks' training algorithm [§2.7] that permits the FFA-ANN with three (3) Neuron Slabs to reach the default error convergence. The grouping of the System's inputs satisfies the approximation of applications' structures and ensures transparency and speed.

The System accepts available inputs and outputs and can extract and use those selected and fed into its next strata. Moreover, it takes under consideration the time evolution of its input vectors by comparing all its partial results (intermediate decisions) before reaching the final decision.

Furthermore, the special System's structure, beyond the employment of hierarchy in input data processing, and therefore its approximation of an expert's "models", makes feasible any project of ANN's development with too many inputs. The separation of inputs into processing stages, from the general knowledge to the specific one, both introduces redundancy in Neurons' number and connections, and ensures, on the other hand, the harmonic disruption of ANNs in parts that can be implemented in hardware and so re-used [6.11].

Within this book's contribution the proposal of a decision support system that is not based on symbolic processing and structuring of its knowledge base's data should also be accounted for. Numeric input, output, and intermediate decision data compose the mapped elements of an application. As a consequence, the novel DSS upholds improved operation speed, transferability to other environments, and digital codification of its data.

2.12 References

[B&C83] Bigger, C. J. and Coupland, J. W., Expert Systems: A Bibliography, IEE Pub., 1983.

[W&K84] Weiss, S. and Kulikowski, C., A Practical Guide to Designining Expert Systems, Rowman and Allanheld, New Jersey, 1984.

[Alt87] Alty, J. L., "The Limitations of Rule Based Expert Systems", Knowledge-Based Expert Systems in Industry, Kriz, J. (editor), pp. 17-22, Ellis Horwood Limited, Chichester, 1987.

[Lip87] Lippmann, R. P., "An Introduction to Computing with NN", IEEE ASSP Mag., vol. 5, pp. 4-22, 1987.

[Mar88] Martorelli, W. P., "PC-Based Expert Systems Arrive", Datamation, vol. 5(4), pp. 56-66, 1988.

[K&P89] Kriketos, B. G. and Pastras, K. S., An Introductory Handbook to Expert Systems, Association for the Development of Nautical Technology, Piraeus, 1989.

[Hil90] Hillman, D. V., "Integrating NN and Expert Systems", AI Expert, vol. 5(6), pp. 54-59, 1990.

[J&F90] Jacob, R. J. K. and Froscher, J. N., "A Software Engineering Methodology for Rule-Based Systems", IEEE Trans. on Knowl. and Data Eng., vol. 2, pp. 173-189, 1990.

[S&T92] Scalero, R. S. and Tepedelenlioglu, N., "A Fast New Algorithm for Training Feedforward NN", IEEE Trans. on Sig. Proc., vol. 40, pp. 202-210, 1992.

[Hay94] Haykin, S., Neural Networks: A Comprehensive Foundation, IEEE Press, 1994.

[E94 I] Economou, G. - P. K., Spiropoulos, K., Economopoulos, N. M., Charokopos, N., Zikos, P., Lymberopoulos, D., and Goutis, C. E., "Decision Supporting Systems in Medical Diseases' Diagnosis: An Artificial Neural Networks Approach", Proc. of Annual Fall Meeting of the Biomedical Society, pp. 123 - 129, Tempe, USA, Oct. 1994.

[E94 II] Economou, G. - P. K., Economopoulos, N. M., Charokopos, N., Zikos, P., Lymberopoulos, D., Spiropoulos, K., and Goutis, C. E., "Suggesting Diagnosis of Diseases and Treatment: How far Artificial Neural Networks can go?", Proc. of 1994 IEEE ISANN, pp. 626 - 631, Tainan, Taiwan, Dec. 1994.

[E95] Economou, G. - P. K., Economopoulos, N. M., Lymberopoulos, D., and C. E. Goutis, "Experiences Accumulated Working towards

Medical Decision Support Systems", J. of Microprocessing and Microprogramming, vol. 40, pp. 883-886, 1995.

3rd Chapter

Medical Decision Support Systems

Let data tell their story...
B. Kosko

3.1 Introduction

The previous chapter presented an original decision support system which was unique in that it was developed by using artificial neural networks. In order for its qualities to be studied in real-life applications, it was first applied in medicine. The reasons ware to gain an insight on: the special difficulties of such a project, the importance of the approach, and a comparison with existing Systems.

Medical Decision Support Systems (MDSSs) are anticipated to provide inference diagnosis engines to both specialized and/or non-medical doctors, to help them on tutoring trainee MDs, and to indicate probable treatments by means of a well-defined flow of intermediate decisions. Furthermore, since MDs ask for and consult a great number of test results, such a specialised Medical System will also take care of these labour intensive tasks. Moreover, MDs who find themselves a long distance away from medical centers have the flexibility of making an estimated diagnosis using MDSSs by accessing data other than from the field that they specialize in. A Medical System performs better in collaboration with the specialist MD and is not an impersonal tool as it is capable to perform adequately in the hands of unskilled users.

Our area of interest was aimed at pulmonary diseases and haematology. Each of these medical fields presents its own particularity and different traits. At the same time, the training Patterns ought to be confirmed by a researcher under more strict rules because of their special importance to their immediate subject - human life.

The above specialties of medicine are dealt with not only as a study environment but also as Systems' application fields, since they are governed by human experience as the main decision factor. The development of a Medical System also should cope with the mistrust with which it is confronted, and also with the non-standardization of the many parameters of the field.

3.2 Decision Support Systems in Medicine

Setting up Medical Systems constitutes a difficult accomplishment. MDSSs require a high-level knowledge of the influences developed between their sub-systems (whose relationships are often non separable), and proper differentiation between conflicting data [Mul90, Pol91, UMS91]. The specialized MD has created, during his/her learning, the necessary coherence so as to distinguish them, while his/her hospital experience enforces his/her knowledge on the pathophysiology of patients.

Such a life experience cannot be enclosed in a set of specific rules and, therefore, is not easily incorporated in computer programs [Pol91].

Patterns with or without special pre-processing (that concern countable data, estimations of parameters, up to attributes' description) are used to form knowledge bases [Ole92], techniques for their representation are developed (that are related to their standardization in reference systems) [Dur93], and it can be said that they are some results - although not entirely those one expects.

Existing Medical Systems require improvements as highlighted in the bibliography. One of its main reasons is related to the variation that characterizes the diseases, in turn this depends on a patient's geographic/topographic area of residence and work, the profession he/she practices, his/her familiar and personal medical file (history data), use of medicines, psychological reasons, etc.

At the same time, diseases' mutations are considered important characteristics in the continuous improvement of Medical Systems. These become evident as the diseases themselves show different symptoms, there are deviations of medical data from the normal value (e.g. fever's intensity), there are demand-improved treatments, and require specialized knowledge for distinguishing and identifying them.

The results of many diseases' superimposition also create difficulties: its results should be classified as multiple diseases and not as a new disease. Should the structure of traditional Systems be applied in medicine, it would be unable to sort through those data [§2.5]. Moreover, the abundance of medical data which accompanies most diseases, creates obstacles in the implementation of MDSSs. These are highlighted by the need for appropriate inductive control techniques, possibly bridging different scientific areas.

These control techniques should satisfy large number of inputs, often supplementing and inter-relating to each other, as it will be shown next. Inputs shall be fed from medical data: symptoms (e.g. wheezing) and their findings (their values, e.g. intensity). Other issues such as the findings' format are related to the man-machine interface and are considered separately.

Each symptom has its own diagnostic merit that can be tracked, described, and exploited with difficulty. Symptoms and their findings evolve in time as a disease develops so that their specific time-related importance can be disregarded by most Medical Systems. As a result, the eventual future visits to the MD are considered as new ones and the integral correlations of all visits' symptoms are indirectly fed to some medical decision support systems.

However, already since 1960, many Medical Systems were proposed, while DSSs, in general, were exploited in the fields of pharmacy [Gor73, S&P78, SBF79, Stu88]. These Medical Systems mostly dealt with the classification of medical data into possible diseases by comparing new data to pre-stored symptoms - their control techniques counting on heuristic and statistical correlations of medical data. They were quickly proved incapable of dealing with the evolution of diseases [Mul90].

More recently, Medical Systems were presented for melanoma detection [Dha88], recovery of the exact extension in incision operations of lymphomas [Kam89], and cases for establishing skin cancer [UMS91]. In all the aforementioned cases, a correct decision critically affects the patient's health, so they will be examined extensively in separate secions [§3.4.1|2|3|4|5].

3.3 Medical Decision Support Systems' Specifications

In the previous chapter, general and specific characteristics for the development of decision support systems were discussed. The way those traits apply to Medicine is the subject of this section, as determined by users, specifications, and the use of ANNs.

3.3.1 The Users' Demands

Generally, medical decision support systems are implemented to application development environments that follow the models of DSSs - as already described [§2.3]. Since medical doctors (MDs) and other users in the medical field do not feel **acquainted** with the field of informatics, computers, and their technology, some reluctance in using MDSSs must first be overcome.

Furthermore, a **friendly environment** is demanded, for a more personal communication interface between man-machine. Medical Systems cannot take the place of the relation between MDs-patients and they must also be adapted to the specialist traits. The **non-standardization** of medical data, just as the sorting and the coding of findings, obstructs the approximation even more. Different teams of doctors face the issue with different communication demands, as it will be shown next.

Moreover, the demand for lower data **processing time** is very important. Modern technological implementations of the hardware and software respond quickly, at least during the use of a Medical System (data processing); quick data supply and faster learning remains to be solved. Usually, data input **consumes** more time than the process itself and in obtaining the results.

The capability to use **incomplete** or **corrupted input vectors** is a major requirement of an MD. Stored medical data rarely ascribe the total condition of patients or provide whole integrated data referring to all the findings of a model medical database. The collaboration with the MD, who usually "codificates" medical data in "keys" for easiness and protection, is necessary. Basic medical data are preferred as specialists create their own way to complete patients' history, thus differentiating "schools" being based on these recordings.

The performance of Medical Systems to an acceptable **reliability degree**, integrates the MD required characteristics. It has to remain high in the diagnosis of new cases and the Medical System should promote intermediate decisions even with small possibility. In this case, the MD is chosen to be the final judge, not the MDSS.

3.3.2 Dynamics of Medical Systems' Development

MDSSs are developed in order to simulate the diagnostic function of specialized medical doctors. They accept and map in their inputs findings, they tend towards the **process model** of MDs, and implement inductive decision mechanisms.

MDDDs satisfy demands such as the **mapping** of medical data and their **storage** in a knowledge base [E95]. This stage is hindered by the non-standardization into a reference base that characterizes them. Features such as colour (appearance, size, skin), seriousness and metrical sizes of findings during their evaluation as causes of diseases (their importance varies among "medical schools"), etc., usually are qualified according to the specialists' perception. Next they are made into inputs, continuous or discrete, binary or not, depending on the necessity.

This mapping often requires **pre-processing** of some or all the available findings. Mapping transformations of colours, images, laboratory examinations' results, etc., are considered necessary for a Medical System that processes this particular kind of data (symbols). These transformations, however, possibly introduce to the System other knowledge odds and ends (i.e. computer numerical accuracy) [Alt87].

The **number** of inputs/outputs, that Medical Systems are called to handle contributes to their complexity. Typically, only for a patient's history, at least two hundred (200) different inputs are required.

The large number of inputs creates problems in the development of knowledge base's **control techniques**. The inputs' participation in the diagnosis of the disease and their processes - so as to institute the inference engine - differs even between MDs of the same specialty. For example, should the explanation of symptoms involving body areas among MDs of different specialties be counted - as well medical "schools" and the diseases mutations - these techniques' need in readjustment is effortless enough only as long as they are arranged for each team of medical doctors, separately.

This readjustment warrants the intervention of the MDs in the Medical System even during the processing of new cases. The processing flow of a MDSS should be such as to facilitate a specialist's possible intervention in order to strengthen some intermediate decisions, according to his/her judgment [§3.8.2].

In previous sections, the importance of DSSs to render a decision **path** with an understandable manner was also highlighted [§2.5]. In order to achieve this goal, a model medical examining procedure for extracting-assessing medical data and for evaluating them should be embodied in the Medical System during its development. Such a model constitutes the **Clinical Differential Diagnosis Methodology** (CDDM) that is arranged in **diagnostic phases**; because of its particular importance all CDDM steps will be developed in section [§3.6].

The **recalling** of medical data from the knowledge base of Medical Systems - so as to provide medical cases that have already been effectively treated - has to be done with great speed. The MD specialists usually choose as their tools "degenerated" Medical Systems, that operate more as quick databases than as inference engines.

Medical decision support systems usually are **limited** in their function by the intended usefulness for which the teams of specialized doctors, who collaborate in their implementation, propose them. Not always obvious, but most MDs look with sceptical disbelief at the establishment of similar technological achievements in their field of expertise. Yet, the MDSS's developer should take in consideration that the willingness of MDs to collaborate decreases greatly while the Medical System is only used for suggestions and not as decisions' support.

Generalization is an expected quality of the Medical System. This is characterised by the need to avoid accessing the same results whether new inputs are processed by such a system or when the system itself is to be used in similar/dissimilar areas of expertise. A successful MDSS is mostly judged by its utilization by the specialized MDs.

MDs will not like to part with a successful MDSS structure even in a different application [UMS91, Dur93], while its effectiveness will permit its propagation in other specialties.

From all the above MDSS characteristics, it is concluded that they have useful results in **limited fields of medicine** [Ole92], or limited to diseases referring to human organs [Kam89, Mul90, Pol91]. A basic purpose of this book was the coverage of an even more extended area of application [E94 I, ..., IV], [E95].

Finally, the development of a DSS in medicine should take under consideration an array of logistical issues or define the application and promotion fields of the final product. Moreover, it should propose the expansion of its use in resembling segments of human experience, not necessarily medical in nature [E95].

3.3.3 Results from the use of Artificial Neural Networks

The decision support system discussed in [§2.9] was applied to the field of medicine and in particular to pulmonary diseases and haematology, as shown next. These Medical Systems, that already fulfil the aforementioned specifications, present also some additional qualities, in relation to the previously presented DSSs.

The more **extensive exploitation** of the entire available medical knowledge, stored in their base, constitutes a key characteristic. The MD usually cannot distinguish the value of major (important) from redundant data and their correlations because of their large numbers. The new Medical System, thanks to its structure and the ANNs [§3.8], undertakes this role and induces data correlations so as to offer even very interesting innovative results [Pol91]. This quality is also confirmed by the remarks of medical teams in relation to making a decision during the development, learning, and the controlling of Medical Systems.

The novel MDSSs also present exploitation of the **entire** available medical knowledge **in each stage** of intermediate and final decisions extraction. The classic DSSs, by means of their inference engine, structure their knowledge base into search or tree graphs [§2.4]. Thus, their stored knowledge is distributed in these branches and the insertion of new inputs is **partially** compared to it. Correlations of medical data and comparison data are exploited only if they were foreseen in their learning or they were known *a priori*. ANNs compare each input with all their Patterns.

The application field of the new Medical System satisfies the demands of the collaborating medical teams and trainee students. MDs can use it as a practice environment to exercise their knowledge. So far, the ascertained **completeness** in its learning (control of the System by the developing teams), the **clarity** in the decisions' extraction (intermediate decisions are collated in each stage), and the **friendliness** in its use (apprehensive decisions' extraction) support this choice.

Experienced MDs, who would need an integrated **second opinion** to make their diagnosis, can use it as a useful tool that correlates present data and its previous learning. Furthermore, MDs who serve long distances from organized medical centers can estimate the seriousness of the diagnosed symptoms on the basis of medical findings even in an area in which they are not specialized.

3.4 Brief Description of Previous Medical Systems

In the next sections some known medical decision support systems are presented for comparative reasons. The problems that they were made to face, and up to a degree solve, and the difficulties in their set-up and development are highlighted. On their whole they have been chosen to cover specific sections of a wide spectrum of medical applications. These sessions refer to modern Medical Systems that are characterized by completeness, integrity and they are arranged expressively depending on the application, the implementation, and their effectiveness.

3.4.1 Finding Elements Displaying the Existence of Gastric Cancer

The greater cause of early death of Japanese citizens is attributed to gastric cancer [Kam89]. Their frenzied life style and the level of technological development make necessary and possible the inspection for gastric tumors even on a daily base. This check up can be carried out in person, while the necessary diagnostic tools are sold in shops.

All things considered, the usual treatment consists mostly in severing the affected sections rather than in administering medications. The MDs enquiry, therefore, is finding the **incision area**, its **surface**, and its **depth** in order to perform the operation.

It can be briefly said that Japanese specialist MDs would look forward to an automated procedure that will eventually correctly promote the above elements - mostly based on previous successful diagnoses, operations, and recoveries. These elements are derived from organized medical databases while the problem's nature (data recall and processing, specifications about operation speed and data evaluation, data identification, etc.) is the lever for the collaboration of different specialists.

The need for quickly finding the correct elements becomes more commanding as the patients-to-be-operated waiting list reaches great numbers. Major goals specifications have been set towards: the systematic **analysis** of all the provided data; the **processing** of a large number of cases; the pursuit for a great rate of **accuracy** in diagnosis; the response **speed** of an appropriate Medical System, and its **friendliness**, since the MDSS will be used mostly by surgeons.

A researchers' team developed a software tool on a personal computer capable of processing 3'843 cases of gastric cancer [Kam89] repeatedly, until the relative data were identified as similar to the patient's. Data were taken from:
- Hospitals' data archives.
- Formal annual government tables.

- Some of their missing data were **statistically completed**.

This program responds in only a few minutes and succeeds in the 96.5% of cases, finding the relatively identical operating data cases.

Inputs to the Medical System are the following:
- Sex of the patient.
- Age of the patient.
- Lymphomatic category of the tumour.
- Invasion's depth of the tumour.
- Location of the tumor. The following occurrences are considered:
  - . Highest, Mean, and Lowest Third of the stomach.
  - . Bigger and Smaller Curvature of the stomach.
  - . Forward and Back Wall of the stomach.
- Diameter of the primary tumour.
- Histological category of the tumour.

This MDSS mainly constitutes a database for the statistical analysis and the recalling of a large number of cases. **Diagnosis is not the issue**, the methodology of confrontation **has been decided** *a priori* (incision) and does not present variations. The inputs and outputs have been mapped to numerical elements so the verification of new cases can be performed with a simple **comparison of the data**.

As the researchers point out, their Medical System does not help in the choice of pharmaceutical or operating treatment, neither can constitute the basis for processing more detailed findings. The large percentage of success in the finding of **statistically identical patient cases** and the limited, however focused, use of the MDSS, were good enough results for the specific period it was utilized. The simplicity of the Medical System also strengthened its practical benefits (i.e. speed).

3.4.2 Finding Elements Displaying the Existence of Dementia

Mulsant invented a medical decision support system for the diagnosis of dementia [Mul90]. His target was to understand the inference engines of artificial neural networks and to be able to present a Network that would converge reliably to such a diagnosis. The difficulty consisted in the difference of the diseases' symptoms as described in the medical and clinical records (lack of findings' standardization between MDs working with, or not, medical centres), as much as in the discovery of the necessary input Patterns for the Medical System's learning.

The entirety of the diseases that are included in this general disease category present medical data as symptoms/findings that:
- Differentiate as long as time elapses.
- Resolve rare cases of generally unknown confrontation with difficulty.
- Barely differentiate from those not related to dementia.
- Correspond to diseases which are cured only if they are identified and confronted in time, with appropriate medical treatment.
- Are identified after long observation.

Moreover, the experience of MDs leads to the diseases' division towards cases that can be successfully treated and are non reversible [Mul90]. This fact, along with, unfortunately, a larger number of the latter, shows that personal factors enter into the classification rates of human experience. This is another factor needing special attention during the development of medical decision support system.

The Medical System was developed on an ANNs basis and a set of heuristic rules developed by the researcher himself. The FFA-ANN was chosen as the architecture of the Network, while the heuristic rules refer to **confidence levels** with which an effort was made to increase the effectiveness of the Medical System. ANNs and heuristic rules co-exist in the structure of the Medical System and only their outputs are compared. The specific Medical System was developed in a workstation environment (IBM RT) and is characterized by:

- 102 inputs that are distributed over 80 medical data and 22 heuristic rules. The heuristic rules are directly mapped to an equal number of outputs.
- 7 outputs-diseases and 22 outputs-questions. The latter are connected directly to the heuristic rules and propose a series of complementary questions for the clarification of a diagnosis. The questions have been decided in advance and are "triggered" (set from the Medical System) after the appropriate combination of input is fed. Essentially, they remind the expert of the **examination procedure** (CDDM).
- 2 Hidden Layers that consist of 10 and 7 Neurons, accordingly. The second Hidden Layer is connected to the 22 outputs-questions by set heuristic rules and to the 7 outputs-diseases by means of Weights.

Furthermore, the Medical System used inputs and outputs where their numerical values were in the close interval [0, 1], implying their position, quality and credibility degree. Also, it was taught by means of the back propagation rule by employing 91 Learning Patterns - 16 of them obtained from MD's experience and the rest were taken from clinical cases. The Patterns were not distributed equally over each disease neither described it in full. Finally, it was tested in 18 new cases, with a success of 77% in relation to the already-given (learnt) diagnoses.

This early study showed good results in relation to the objective difficulty of the problem. The fact that ANNs can be used for the mapping of the incoming medical data is again highlighted in an application that can be said is ruled by criteria less objective; personal observations lead the diagnosis.

The use of expert (heuristic) rules to boost the Medical System's credibility indicates the "controversy" of ANN's use in a field that **is not constrained by specific classification criteria**. On the other hand, the **small number** of Learning Patterns and its **non-balanced use** during learning, imposed to the Network, does not totally ensure the conditions of an equally distributed hyperspace classification [§1.3]. It makes up, however, a very good development base of more inspired medical decision support systems that should use more Patterns and should be fed with more strict criteria or categories' examples.

3.4.3 Finding Elements Displaying the Existence of Hypertension

A team of researchers have tried to identify the problem of diagnosis and proper treatment of hypertension [Pol91]. It is a heart disorder that appears in 15-20% of the population and can cause serious heart arrhythmias, chronic exhaustion or other fatal diseases.

The team developed a simulation model of a Medical System capable of distinguish the existence of the disease based on recoded high blood pressure – the only known cause for its manifestation. The model was also constructed to provide the appropriate medical treatment. ANNs again formed the basis of the system, which was divided into the following subsystems:
- The reference-generating module that responds according to and compares the blood pressure of patients and healthy people of the same sex and age. The measurements covered a twenty-four hours period - one per each hour. Where medical data were not known, **an expert average value of the unknown one was given** so that the Medical System was taught with complete Patterns.
- The corresponding drug module examined **drug compatibility** and suggested the type of medicine that will benefit the patient without the added irritation of any known side effects.
- The therapy-selecting module proposed the final **prescription** of the medications and their dosage.

The first module consists of 2 three-level Networks (with 1 Hidden Layer), of FFA-ANN type. One of these levels was taught by using the age and the sex of a healthy human while the other accomplishes the same classification but for patients. They respond by giving the corresponding references of blood pressure by using:
- 2 inputs.
- 4 Neurons in their Hidden Layer.
- 24 outputs, one for each hour.

The second module, also of FFA-ANN type, consists of 2 layers with 17 input-data that depict medical human classes and 4 outputs-categories of medications.

The third module, of FFA-ANN type as well, constitutes the main body of the medical decision support system. It accepts the outputs of the previous subsystems and responds with the medications dosage. This ANN presents special characteristics as it contains:
- 58 inputs that correspond to:
  . 24 inputs-differences of the Systolic Blood Pressure values between patients and healthy people.
  . 24 inputs-differences of the Diastolic Blood Pressure values between patients and healthy people.
  . 6 clinical findings.
  . the 4 outputs of the second module
- 4 Hidden Layers, of 12 Neurons each in order that:
  . the first correlates the results of the differences between patients-healthy people based on the blood pressure categories.
  . the second correlates the outputs of the first Hidden Layer and the medical data that arise from the clinical files.
  . the third correlates the outputs of the second Hidden Layer and the data that arise from the second subsystem.

- the fourth depicts the results of the third Hidden Layer in the ANN's output (that is also the Medical System's output).
- 96 outputs that indicate the allowance of each of the 4 medication categories per hour in a daily period of time.

The ANNs were submitted to the back propagation rule and in a different number of Learning Patterns each. Precisely, records of 200 patients of mixed sex and age between 20-80 years were fed in the ANNs of the first module. The Learning Period converged to a little number of Synapses, not achieving memorization but correlation of all data with which it was taught. As a result, it discovered a **phase shift** in the measurements and an **increase** of the blood pressure depending on the age - elements that **were not statistically found** [Pol91].

The second module was fed with 30 cases of patients and 30 cases of healthy people. The function of this simple Network was proven by means of 10 cases of patients and 10 cases of healthy people and reached 100% correct response rate.

The third module was inputted with 60 records of both patients healthy people. The learning time for the specific Network reached 50 hours. Its response was tested by means of Learning Patterns consisting of 10 healthy people and 25 possible patient cases. It managed to classify:
- 11 input patients in need of treatment - making 1 error.
- 22 input patients as healthy - making 1 error.
- Correct responses with a total accuracy rate of 94%.

In conclusion, this Medical System achieved its limited targets. It succeeded to promote even the medical treatment of the probable patients, but **after being guided** in the choice of limited medication categories. Its general-type architecture permits easy adaptation to similar problems on a small scale.

Despite the abundance of Learning Patterns - that were not completely integral ones - it achieved only a **binary-response logic** resulting in the existence, or not, of **one and only disease**. Moreover, the mapping of the Hidden Layer of the third modules in only specific Neurons, downgrades the use of an ANN in a look-up table (obligatory projections), without permitting the larger input data correlation; therefore, the creation of inner rules have not been anticipated.

Finally, the case of **partial Learning Patterns** is faced rather loosely and the effect of probable computational error in their development is solved to some extent with the delimitation of their values. This Medical System though, constitutes a robust and elegant solution, a confrontation example of a well defined, partial (sub)problem which requires higher development [Pol91].

3.4.4 Finding Elements Displaying a Distinction between Malignant Tumours
The differentiation between 2 types of malignant tumours of the breast - the tubular carcinoma and the sclerosis adenosis - was the subject of this study [Ole92]. Although biologically they do not resemble each other, their identification processing is obstructed by their similar histological identity.

On the other hand, **statistical methodologies** are difficultly applied as the medical data fall short of normalization and standardization methods when gathering and processing human expertise. Moreover, the specialized MDs (who achieve the identification of patterns) do not manage to **metrically** depict their knowledge. There is a constant argument on the inserted rate, the kind, and the results by the **measurements noise**. In total, the only acceptable comparative model presupposes the morphologic, stereological, and modular examination of these tumours. The last, though, carries the danger of the tumour inflammation towards fatal cancer.

By using 18 tumour patterns for each one of their types, 18 measurements of their stereological and morphologic natures (shape and size mainly) were taken. Specialized MDs classified these measurements, which were fed in 1 FFA-ANN of 3 layers of full connected Neurons. The back propagation rule was chosen as the learning algorithm and the ANN converged to yield the following results:
- After the use of two logical levels ("0", "1") for their I/O pairs.
- During the completion of 460'000 Learning Cycles.
- With a rate of 92% in the identification of its Patterns.

Correspondingly, when it was fed with 19 novel Test Patterns, it presented 100% classification accuracy. As a conclusion, the results were judged as satisfying and the ANNs further learning was terminated.

In short, the experiment was more based on the appropriate **pre-processing** of Patterns than on the physiology of the diagnosis. The researchers also focused on the presentation of an acceptable model for tumours study and the appropriate reasoning concerning the use of ANN. Their chosen Network gathered many interesting features, but its learning and use have some disadvantages.

The ANN does not classify neither inducts diagnoses but rather acts as a **quick memory for data recall**. The disability of not exploiting statistical methods properly is being bypassed, but the number of input Patterns was not large. The researchers themselves highlight its inability to indicate as irrelevant input Patterns that do not belong to any of the two tumours categories.

3.4.5 Finding Elements Displaying the Existence of Malignant Melanoma

In the United States of America the prevention and cure of malignant melanoma has the largest medical public awareness of any disease. Amongst all kinds of skin cancer, it has the higher attack rate in the least time. The high fatality rate and the way of life of this country's inhabitants, in combination with the ozone's hole and the devastating impact of the sun's ultraviolet radiation, does render its early diagnosis of utmost importance [Dur93].

The researching team first [UMS91] tried to set-up a method to increase the melanoma's diagnostic accuracy by utilizing pre-processed input data taken from images and the use of ANNs. By achieving a large percentage of correct diagnosis, especially on the primary stages of the disease, the patient undertakes a biopsy examination of the tumour and afterwards, an operation for its extraction. The problem when using this examination is the possibility of benign tumours being converted into malignant ones. At the same time, the operation for the extraction of the tumour, especially in far-gone stages, does not secure the patient.

First, 2 specific type Medical Systems were implemented, being based on shape, colour, and size data extracted by the use of special algorithms. One of them exploited the inductive algorithm ID3 and the other one heuristic rules. Their effectiveness rated within a range of 86-92% and 26-78%, respectively. Other numerical methods used by the team gave an accuracy of 62-65%.

The recently published Medical System [Dur93] is composed of a separate inspector controlling the outputs of multiple three-level ANNs of restricted Coulomb energy type. The feeding of a novel Pattern to such an ANN, during the learning period, simulates the supply of a positive electrostatic ion into a negative charged field. The storage of the Pattern in this ANN is performed by means of appropriate Weights between its I/O connections and by utilizing specific Hidden Layers of Neurons. Its learning algorithm ensures the local differentiation of the Neural memory in each insertion of a novel Pattern.

The final system - comprising of separate inspector and the ANN – was named Nestoras, after the wise Homeric character of the Iliad.

The standardization of the input data proved to be a major task. Different methods for a series of processes that would bring in numerical values were used, such as:
- Image segmentation, so the region of interest can to be extracted from it.
- Its chromatic transformation, so that specific colours can be highlighted. These colours were chosen after the suggestion of an experts' team.
- Feature extraction from input data such as:
  . Shape.
  . Edges.
  . Texture.
  . Crust.
  . Hair.
- Colour normalization based on the patient's skin. It was proven that this factor enhanced the performance of whatever method used.
- Surface and depth of the tumour (wherever possible), although the actual numbers were not used but rather their normalized values versus known tumours.

The medical decision support system was fed by means of:
- 18 inputs
- Processing data after 250 pictures of melanomas.
- The use of two logical levels ("0", "1").

The pictures were separated in a large number of sets that, in turn, were used for learning and generalizing purposes (divisions of 10%, 20%, …, 80%, 90%). With this methodology the compatibility in learning was ensured, with regards to the previous efforts - as the methods' comparison was also an issue.

Nestoras' performance achieved a level of 80% of correct diagnoses. This percentage was achieved for the largest set of Learning Patterns, something that was also generally observed within the previous efforts. More specifically, Nestoras predominated over other methods when taught with the smaller sets of Patterns, and fell short when it was taught on the larger ones.

The aims of the research were not completely covered. Explicit results regarding the various methodologies' effectiveness were not clear - neither important accurate diagnosis was established. The researchers believe that the psychophysiology of human vision must evolve more to achieve the full exploitation of the images' data. Also, medicine must progress on finding the melanoma's origins.

On the other hand, Nestoras exploited its ANNs as classifiers-comparators. Researchers usually put aside the importance of human senses when treating findings in lieu of a statistical, metrical, robust, approximate pre-processing of them; such findings do not enforce the results obtained biologically. The Learning Patterns, also, were only concerned with pre-processed data. Finally, the feeding of negative models could be more appropriate in this case (i.e. a clearer explanation of what a skin tumour is, so that this will not be confused with a melanoma).

3.5 Conclusions Gathered from the Use of Previous Medical Systems

The aforementioned Medical Systems have also shown some intrinsic disadvantages, mostly because they were not created as applications for general purposes. They constitute very a good implementation of decision support systems with relatively good response to new input data but with intense specialization.

Generally, they use **data pre-processing** before the utilization of mapping and representation techniques in learning algorithms. Special purpose algorithms were developed for the extraction of useful data from the medical ones by adding, however, the computational error of each one. The expertise of other fields' experts, that is also inserted in the Medical System, constitutes an inhibiting factor for their application, as it includes other elements and sets necessary for the presence of all the specialists during the modifications of the MDSS.

On the other hand, they refer to disease cases that **specifically affect only some organs of the body**. Also, all the diseases affecting those organs are neither covered nor stand as integral examples of all medical cases.

At the same time, they are presented as **inflexible**, adapted only to the applications for which they were developed. With great difficulty, they manage to augment their knowledge bases, expand with their adaptation to other applications, or cover other diagnostic fields. The exploitation of their capabilities is generally non-profitable, as their vast cohesion with the area they cover signifies the utilization of some of its unique characteristics - generally a feature hard to find in other cases.

A "spirit" of **prejudice** also accompanies them and other teams of MDs seldom use them if they did not participate themselves in their development. The same spirit also obstructs the more **general collaboration** of specialists from many scientific areas. The combined collaboration usually constitutes an impossible task; however, many scientific articles highlight its advantages.

In order to target the development of productive and reliable Medical Systems, the well-established collaboration base of all the related experts must be a necessity. The level of satisfaction in the correct application, function, and standardization of these decision support systems depends on the link amongst the specialists in each area – this also affects the viability. The medical knowledge and experience presupposes absolute experts' attention, as it copes with human lives. Finally, bringing together different experts' aspects may lead to even more erros - independently of the MDSS application field.

As a consequence, artificial intelligence techniques are forwarded on modern Medical Systems, so the convergence on the medical way of thinking and MDs experience become an asset [B&S84, SPS87]. Applications of such techniques and of Medical Systems are continually generalized, covering fields that traditionally analysed the ability of human thought and apprehension [Mul90].

These techniques mainly embody methodologies that try to emulate the human way of **perception and understanding**, the **logical consequence**, and the actual **reasoning** with reference to the control techniques. The problem, which is related to the performance of the specialized experience, always exists. Many cases are reported where the MD simply "had an intuition".

Moreover, artificial intelligence techniques incorporate the estimation and evaluation of new data, which are continually discovered. Finally, they carefully approach the conclusions and the decisions which are based on Learning Patterns and control techniques, and which are developed in parallel with the application.

Although they collaborate with each other, they contradistinguish the **classic algorithms** of: the "if... then... else" scenarios, the serial programming, and the serial techniques of discovery and register, by implementing Medical Systems that learn with the use of examples (input-output data). Deductively, they are similar to known rules of thumb and heuristic practices that are acquired during the continuous occupation of an object and are rarely transferred by the use of standards.

Artificial intelligence techniques are exploited either for the achievement of a special inference engine methodology of DSSs, or as the means for the realization of both the knowledge base and the **induced decision procedure** [UMS91, Hen92, Dur93]. The last is defined as the composition of a general purpose System from a set of examples that cover the entire examined field so as to operate as the optimum classifier with a clear flow of decisions for each output. Generally, it can be said that their performance is judged productive and better than that of Systems that are developed from the classic programming methods. On the other hand, their typical disadvantages also stand - even to a smaller degree.

3.6 Clinical Differential Diagnosis Methodology

In medicine, by "diagnosis" we mean: the name of the patient's disease, the condition of the deteriorated function of an organism, and the examining procedure for the determination of his/her health status. When applying the medical clinical differential diagnosis methodology, an MD uses a speculative procedure that is many times re-iterated, and comprises many **diagnostic phases**. These form a model estimation of the findings, inductive thought, and decision [DeG81].

By means of these diagnostic phases, the MD gathers and estimates the diseases' signs. The diagnostic phases are 4, namely:
- Phase 1: Understanding of medical events.
- Phase 2: Assessment of medical events.
- Phase 3: Drawing out a series of assumptions.
- Phase 4: Selection between assumptions.

3.6.1 Understanding of Medical Events

By means of a "train of questions" between a specialized MD and a patient, the first is informed about medical data like the patient's own personal history, his symptoms (i.e. "Fever") or findings (i.e. "Temperature"), and the time elapsed since they became evident. The **symptomatology**, as a term, is referred to their evaluation. The elements taken from such a conversation, are the **subjective** data of an MD's examination (since they are derived from a patient). These "subjective" elements are usually compared with the official medical history of the patient and they vary thematically depending on the MD specialization [DeG81].

Next, the MD performs a series of physical examinations, namely the **objective** data [DeG81]. These objectives are plotted against subjective data to confirm or reject the physical examination (due to a patient's failure to describe his/her condition properly).

The physical examinations fall into one of the following general categories and remain identical to or are adapted from them, depending on the MD specialization:
- Auscultation.
- Percussion.
- Inspection.
- Palpation.

3.6.2 Assessment of Medical Events

The contradistinction of the "objective" versus the "subjective" data, of an MD's examination, is performed at the same time as their comparison with the normal values (those of a health human, similar to a patient's medical type). The medical data that most concern the MD, depending on his/her specialization, are gathered and then archived according to his/her experience and habits.

3.6.3 Drawing Out a Series of Assumptions

After taking into account all the gathered medical events, the MD is called to decide how these are combined in order to indicate categories and diseases. According to his/her experience or by resorting to already-compiled reference catalogues, he/she creates lists of medical elements and their corresponding symptoms and findings for each disease that falls into his/her expertise. In this way, **guiding points,** variable in number and importance, are created ready to indicate possible diseases [DeG81].

3.6.4 Selection between Assumptions

This stage is the core of the medical differential diagnosis and proposes the independent, gradual evaluation of all medical data, their findings, symptoms, and assessment and decisions concerning diseases. Each category of diseases and each separate disease are examined in turn, and their indications made to intersect with the patient's important indications (decided in advance).

According to the CDDM, i.e. while comparing points (experience) and elements (medical data), the sparing rule is applied following which, from the initial list, one and only one disease must result. Despite this rule, though, "there are not diseases but patients" and as a consequence the specialized MDs do not discard any disease until they establish the final diagnosis. Keeping this in mind, they create a second list with ensuing laboratory examinations, the results of which will exercise the higher weight in reaching the final decision (diagnosis) [DeG81].

The phases of the CDDM are complementary and usually an MD resorts to them retrospectively, continually, and in different times after the patient's first examination. Deductively, the most important factor for the development of medical decision support systems based on the CDDM constitutes the management's independence in the inspection of points and elements.

3.7 Medical Examination Using the Novel Medical System

The 4 phases of the clinical differential diagnosis methodology were incorporated in the novel Medical System. This should achieve a great standardization level in reaching a decision and the "path" that is followed for its extraction - to make sense to the MD. The basic points, that were applied for its incorporation, follow:
- Each medical datum (element, symptom, or finding) is individually examined.
- No conclusions on a patient's condition should be reached before all available medical data of him/her have been gathered and evaluated. The findings of the examination must be considered apart from each other.
- Medical data processing should lead from more general to more specific conclusions; this rule applies to both the symptomatology and the diagnosis.

The novel Medical System is based on many independent ANNs and is implemented by a model architecture that utilizes **four levels of Networks** and to each medical major medical data (i.e. each symptom) corresponds an ANN, thus structuring the (initial) **Level #1** (Fig. 2.3 and Fig. 3.2). Each Network has as many inputs as the number of findings of the proper medical datum, and responds either with the categories or the diseases. At the same Level, similar ANNs will be fed by a patient's physical examinations results.

Level #2 of the novel MDSS's ANNs accept the outputs of the Level #1 and combines them in pairs of two with the physical examinations' ANNs output. Furthermore, it extracts categories and diseases. By this, the "subjective" elements of the CDDM "are clarified" while compared with the "objective" ones, as soon as the value of each finding has been considered separately. Therefore, the "re-iteration" of the reasoning - the gathered data correlation - is being performed.

In **Level #3**, composed by one ANN, the results of the previous Networks are supplied to its inputs and the final classification, either possible categories or the diseases, is being "decided". However, no possible decision is discarded by the Medical System since only the MD can decide what data to keep, based on his/her previous medical case expertise.

Level #4 of the medical decision support system consists of one ANN, and proposes laboratory examinations based on the final classification of the categories and diseases, thus finalizing the first decision support (diagnosis cycle). The MDSS's operation is detailed extensively in the next sections.

3.8 Application of the Novel Medical System to Pulmonary Diseases

A MDSS in the field of pulmonary diseases was developed after the sudden increase in the number of **tuberculosis** and **lung cancer** cases during the last years [E94 IV]. Artificial neural networks constitute the most appropriate selection for the development of a Medical System, as the nature of pulmonary data is characterized by complexity.

Multiple dependencies between all medical elements are dominant and still undefined even by specialized MDs. The ANNs exploit all existing relations, the ones that the MD suggests and those he/she applies without being able to express them consciously; the latter are fed by means of Learning Patterns.

Incomplete input vectors, i.e. medical data forming those Patterns also portray pulmonary diseases. As it is shown in Table 3.1, the proper coverage of the reference space presupposes a plethora of inputs. Naturally, all these medical data can indicate even remote cases, but they must be known to the ANN so as to contain the whole area. Also, the demand for **correct differentiation** between the given medical data and the overlapping symptoms of different diseases, show the special attributes of the pulmonary data. The ANNs are able to ensure it, based on their classifying abilities.

In order to structure a suitable Medical System, a number of parameters had to be defined [§3.2]. They deal with the feeding of medical data, the wanted induction course, i.e. a methodology for forwarding a result, even without 'being able' to 'tell how', and the selection of the correct architecture and learning algorithm for the ANN under study. This model of a medical decision support system represents the experience of a pulmonologist and is developed separately for each specialized MD.

These parameters were judged necessary so that a **user friendly interface** between the MD and the Medical System (findings' appearance, decision flow selections, intervention of the MD, etc.), the wanted **reliability degree** (that was set at least on the already-examined Medical Systems' level), and the future **utilization** of the final product by the collaborating medical team can be achieved. Under these conditions, the Medical System would evolve, expand and be well exploited.

3.8.1 Grouping of Pulmonary Medical Data

The creation of Medical Systems follows a tedious procedure because of the different emphasis that the various medical "schools" convey to symptoms and findings. "Schools" often vary both on a diagnostic method and proposed treatment. ANNs constitute, again, a very good research selection as they permit an evaluation grading and can employ the most suitable CDDM [§3.8.2]. They can be taught to grant unlikely values to their input, so stressing their output components [4.4].

Specialized MDs of the Pulmonary Department of the Regional University Hospital of Patras, Greece, have set the specifications for a novel Medical System. A specific number of questions - the same ones that are used during the actual

patient's examination - were mapped to the MDSS's inputs. They refer to the following medical data (symptoms, etc.) and their findings:
- Cough, 16 findings.
- Fever, 11 findings.
- Chest Pain, 8 findings.
- Haemoptysis, 5 findings.
- Dyspnoea, 14 findings.
- Wheezing, 9 findings.
- Expectorations, 12 findings.

In addition, medical data were also included in relation to:
- Age, sex, profession, smoking history, appearance of a patient.
- Previous pulmonary diseases.
- Other diseases.
- Receiving of medicines.
- Family history data.

Also included were findings taken from physical examinations:
- Auscultation, 22 findings.
- Percussion, 3 findings.
- Inspection, 10 findings.
- Palpation, 3 findings.

The above are given in alphabetical and not by order of their importance. The novel Medical System had to ponder over 113 inputs, without counting the number of history data findings. The latter amount to 250 inputs.

The Medical System was fed with a Learning Patterns hybrid set that came from theoretical medical knowledge (books, essays, articles), the Hospital MDs team's experience, and the actual medical data regarding 200 files of patient cases; those patients were cured.

These Patterns development was preferred so to favour the **uniform distribution** of findings per disease [§1.3]. This key distribution could not be ensured by the sole utilization of the medical data gathered from the clinical files. This fact introduces another evaluation point about Medical Systems: the importance of the **geographic region** when they weigh up new cases should they have been taught by patients' files only. The collaboration with other MDs is a key factor for the proper generalization.

By means of the use of these Patterns, the **experience of the medical team** is fully exploited; this is not restrained only to MDs' interaction with actual patients but it has been also built up during the MDs training (basic and towards specialization). Mainly, these elements are not necessarily part of patients' files.

Also, it was decided that the novel Medical System ought to cover the **whole spectrum** of the pulmonary diseases, including unknown cases in Greece. In other words, theoretical knowledge had to be fed into the Medical System too. In addition, it is a well-known fact that by only using the patients' clinical files the uniform distribution of diseases is not ensured; theoretical knowledge also bridged this gap.

In conclusion, a rate of 140 out of the 200 actual medical cases were used in the ANNs' learning. The remaining 60 were alternatively used for examining the accuracy of the Medical System when left to generalize [§3.8.3]. As customary, sets of learning/test cases were formed and comparative experiments were conducted.

During the teaching of the Networks, 3 logical levels of input data were used to map the findings' existence [Mul90]:
- **Logical "1"**, indicating the existence of a specific medical data, symptom, or finding, categories or diseases. Logical "1"s are as many for a given Learning I/O Pattern pair as given input and/or output components dictate.
- **Logical "0"**, indicating the non-existence of the above data.
- **Logical "0.5"**, indicating ignorance or indifference about the existence or not of the above. The utilization of this level is qualitatively different from the corresponding one in the aforementioned bibliography [§4.4]. Also, the fact that numerically this logical level is put in the middle of the other two, permits the ANNs to respond after considering probable, additional Learning Pattern characteristics.

This mapping ensures the use of even older, not completed medical files, the mapping of logical levels (and numerical values) to each component of input vectors [3.3.2], and the better evaluation of the ANN's qualities [§4.4], so important **data correlation** [§1.11, §4.2] can be achieved. Furthermore, for the first time, the following learning methodology was adopted:
- Each finding was considered as **self-existent** and was inserted separately in whatever input component was existent (as a logical "1") and by keeping the remaining input components on ignorance status (logical "0.5"). The non-existence of input components was similarly mapped (logical "0").

In this way, the Medical System was taught to learn "positive" and "negative" Patterns thus separate the existence and the non-existence of inputs [§4.5].
- The gravity of the existence or non-existence of some input components in the Patterns was highlighted by the use of factors of **particular data weight**, thus easily focusing on some of them since they were so differentiated.
- Each Learning Pattern has the same number of components (given the logical values) with any other for the same Network, so asymmetries that arise during the creation or the classification of sub-areas will be wiped out. Hence, **pseudo-inputs** (dummy inputs) are used and the asymmetries are now set due to the learnt **Weights**.

Main directions, such as the importance of medical data in a disease's diagnosis, diseases' interaction and the classification of ANNs outputs, were left for the artificial neural networks to be defined. On the other hand, medical data that can indicate the existence or non-existence of fatal diseases were specially considered, utilized, and standardized, so as to have a dominant role.

During the MDSS learning process by means of the analysed **selective feedback procedure**, the Learning Patterns were altered (completed or re-defined) when it was judged necessary by the team of pulmonologists. Thus, the learning time period for the Medical System stretched over a period of 10 months.

Many of the above elements constitute novel ideas in the field of FFA-ANN's learning. The contents of the present chapter are not focused on this learning: however, **data feeding, Learning Patterns' formation**, and the **ANNs' learning** will be the subject of detailed analysis in the next chapter [§4.3|4|6|7|8].

3.8.2 Architecture of the Pulmonary Medical System

The integration of the CDDM in the structure of the novel Medical System was estimated to demand 3 **Layers** of ANNs' arrangements. Each Layer is composed of **Levels** of similarly organized and taught FFA-ANNs that operate based on the principles developed in the previous chapter [§2.9].

The individual ANNs "communicate" only through their outputs, by means of connections that remind those of Neurons in the FFA-ANN. Only the ANNs' results are aggregated so as to supply the final diagnosis. It is the first time that such a scalable DSS's architecture, based in ANNs, was attempted [E94 I-IV], [E95].

Fig. 3.1 represents the aforesaid architecture. It is similar to that shown in Fig. 2.3 and adapted so as to fulfil the demands of the medical decision support system.

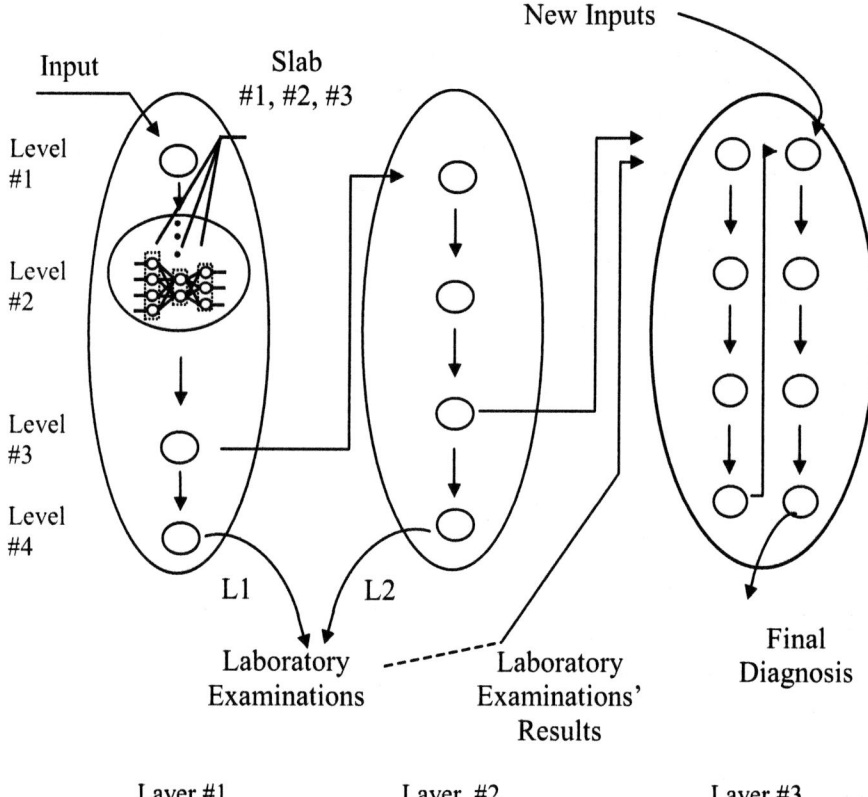

Figure 3.1: Architecture of the Novel Medical Decision Support System

It is important for the reader to notice that Layer #1 promotes its outputs and its successive Networks categories of pulmonary diseases, while Layer #2 the diseases; Layer #3 takes under consideration the results of the laboratory examinations. The graph shown in Fig. 3.2 presents the detailed contents of Layer #1 and generally describes the architecture of the remaining layers.

Layer #1 is composed of 4 Levels of inductive decisions' extraction (Fig. 3.1). It accepts as inputs the findings of the 7 pulmonary symptoms, history data, and of the 4 physical examinations in separate FFA-ANNs. In the place of these findings other organized inputs of whatever other area of interest could well be set if they can be gathered by the application area's structures.

The finding-inputs are combined independently and each of Layers #1, #2, and #3 responds with compatibility ratings (percentage) of the new inputs versus the 13 categories of the pulmonary diseases (Table 3.1). The ratings are not referred as similarity ones (measured by whatever norm [§1.3]), due to the nature of the weights the ANNs developed (due to the special Learning Patterns). As was already mentioned, MDs asked for Layer #1 to output categories of diseases. Yet, Level #4 proposes laboratory examinations from a total of 15 possible ones.

The 9 FFA-ANNs of Level #1 are composed of 3 Slabs [§1.2] each. Experiments confirmed the sufficiency of using only one hidden layer as the wanted learning accuracy was achieved. The one FFA-ANN of Level #4, where the final aggregation between intermediate decisions is actualised, is composed of 2 Slabs.

FFA-ANNs of Levels #2 and #3 (8 and 1 respectively), correlate the intermediate decisions. As stated by the CDDM, on Level #2, the responses of the FFA-ANNs of Level #1 (7 lists of categories of diseases for medical symptoms, plus the one of the history data), are each separately combined to the results of the FFA-ANN of the physical examinations [E94 I-IV]. Level #3 finally correlates all these responses. Level #4 promotes resultant laboratory examinations on a first-level basis (L1).

Layer #2's structure and number of FFA-ANNs are similar to Layer #1's. Still, all Levels of this Layer respond in rates of diseases appropriateness (rather than their categories). Also, this layer's Level #4 promotes resultant laboratory examinations being based on the resulting diseases' classification second-level basis (L2).

Pulmonary diseases sum up to 35 distinct ones, while the response of the last Level of Layer #2 is mainly exploited in Layer #3. Furthermore, each FFA-ANN accepts 13 inputs more than the respective Networks of Layer #1, i.e. the final categories of diseases classification list of the previous Layer (Fig. 3.1).

Layer #3 is composed of two, identical in structure, sets of Levels that are analogous to the corresponding units of Layer #2. The advantage of this structure lies in the simultaneous process and comparison of the patients' medical data and findings - before and after the laboratory examinations. More specifically, more often than not, the slow rate of these examinations' completion and the possible modifications of the medical symptoms that the patients may present during this time, are findings that need to be fed in the novel Medical System separately.

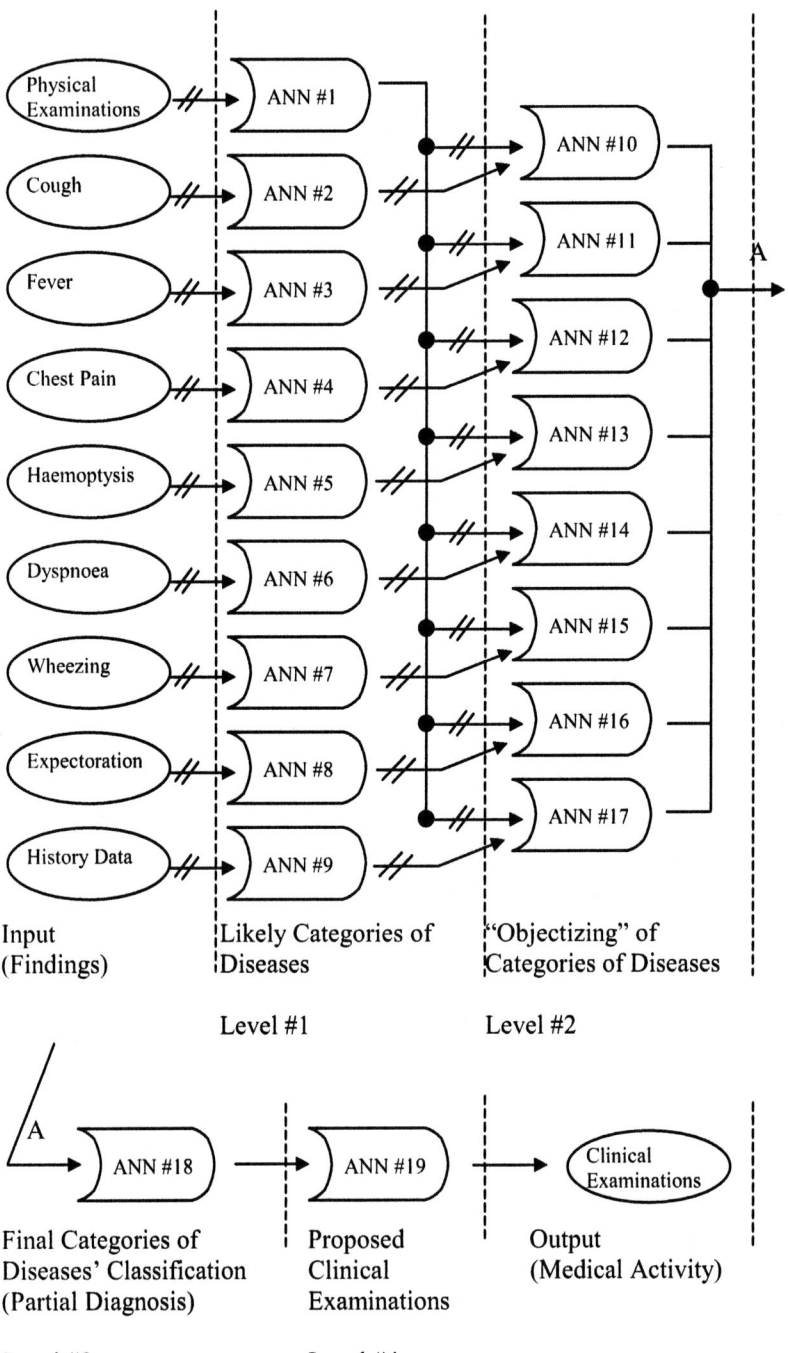

Figure 3.2: Schematic Representation of Layer #1

Layer #3 also receives the results of the laboratory examinations, thus extracting the final diagnosis, the appropriate category(ies) of medicines (selections are done between five medicine "families") and their daily dosage. The necessary Patterns are constantly being enriched with data from specialized pulmonary teams.

Typical learning parameters of the FFA-ANNs include:
- Learning time that rated between 10 and 20 minutes.
- Convergence in 2'000 to 3'000 Learning Cycles.
- Medical System's final response between 2 to 3 minutes.

MDs' verdict pronounced that the set specifications for the MDSS are covered by the above architecture. The FFA-ANNs constitute organized inductive structures that promote a decision from the more general to the more specific data: at the same time, and in such a way, that a probable intervention (by a specialist) can take place in all the intermediate stages they are linked to.

The diagnosis' leading points [§3.6.3] are suitably highlighted during the Networks learning (by means of proper Patterns) and also **during** the decision extraction, since an MD, during the System's operation, is able to change some medical data and intermediate decisions to promote a better fit. Throughout the induction chain, to the final decision, all classifications of diseases are stored so that an MD is able to, at any time, define a decision extraction way that was not anticipated (i.e. building various diagnostic scenarios).

One more element of originality is the comparison of the diagnostic phases before and after the laboratory examinations and the exploitation of the entire experience, stored per each FFA-ANN, during the extraction of the intermediate decision, and not per a specific path of "firing" Networks. The Networks will place the novel input vectors as close as possible to the output Patterns with which they have been taught - as soon as they will have "studied" thoroughly and completely all the Synapses and their intermediate connections. Due to the MDSS specific architecture, this procedure flow demands very little time.

Table 3.1 depicts the symptom "Wheezing" and its findings represent the typical inputs of an FFA-ANN. It should be noticed that some findings overlap while they are mutually shunning each other; however, this does not constitute a paradox. First, such events have been taken care of during the learning; on the other hand, a disease manifests in different temporal phases, so inserting a differentiation.

Also, for the architecture of the Medical System, the key point is that it provides **clarity** in all the units' intermediate results. Consequently, it can back-up whichever final decision (diagnosis) is reached. Moreover, it **does not reject any disease's case (category)** - not even those of small appropriateness. In this way, the final decision is left in the MD's experience although, if requested, it can be provided too.

Through the additional inputs that are accepted by Layer #2 and by the comparison of diagnoses before and after the laboratory examinations in Layer #3, a powerful **amplification** of the System's decision procedure is achieved. According to the associating experimental results before and after the use of both, their combined application lead to a 15% - 25% of improved final decisions' accuracy.

The first Slabs of each FFA-ANN process, through their Sigmoids, the MDSS inputs and prepare them for the second Slabs. Those weigh, aggregate, and forward them, by their Sigmoids again, on the third Slabs. The latter, by means of the same procedure, provide for the FFA-ANNs outputs. Therefore, the second (hidden) Slab is the most important when utilizing FFA-ANNs. Improving a Network's accuracy by increasing the width of this Slab (number of hidden Slabs or Neurons) has not succeeded, mainly because of the **present medical data mapping sufficiency**.

	1	2	3	4	5	6	7	8	9
i									
ii									
iii									
iv(**)	*	*		*			*	*	
v(****)	*	*	*	*	*	*	***	*	
vi(**)		*	*	*	*	*		*	
vii(**)		*	*	*	*			*	
viii(**)			*	*	*	*		*	
ix(**)	*	*	*	*	*		*	*	
x(*)			*		*				
xi									
xii									
xiii(***)	*	*	*	*	*	*		*	*

Respiratorial Deficiency:	i	Recently Exhibited:	1
Abnormalities of the Diaphragm:	ii	Acute:	2
Abnormalities of the Chest Wall:	iii	Periodical:	3
Disorders of the Mediastinum:	iv	Small Duration:	4
Bronchial Asthma:	v	Medium Duration:	5
Interstitial Diseases of the Lungs:	vi	Long Duration:	6
Disorders of the Pulmonary Circulation:	vii	when Inhaling:	7
Occupational Disorders of the Lung:	viii	when Exhaling:	8
Cancer of the Lungs:	ix	Chronic:	9
Infection Diseases of the Lungs:	x		
Disorders of Pleura:	xi		
Tuberculosis-TBC:	xii		
Chronic Obtrusive Pulmonary Disease-COPD:	xiii		

Table 3.1: Wheezing Findings per Category of Pulmonary Diseases

The asterisk (*) is used to denote the significance of a particular medical datum (symptom or finding) to a category of diseases

Thanks to the clarity of the intermediate results throughout all Layers, **alternative diagnoses** can be provided. MDs may judge what medical data are more important per case, according to their experience, and subsequently intervene in the final decision by means of changing the importance of individual data.

The conducted experiments rated the performance of this Medical System between 88% and 95% when left to generalize into new (unknown) inputs and without utilizing any laboratory examinations results. It must not be however assumed that in the rest of the cases (5% - 12%) the System fails. The MD having at his/her service all the System's decision flow, can always redefine the succession of diseases, decide alone, or to input more medical data.

Moreover, by the full exploitation of the laboratory examinations results and the application of new ones, the MDSS' performance is expected to rise. According to the MDs, these examinations provided no doubts on the diagnostic accuracy is of any value. The symptoms' ability to indicate a disease is decreased by the recommended medicines. Finally, it must be noted that the utilized patients' files often did not include laboratory examinations, thus creating ambiguity.

3.8.3 Control and Exploitation of the Pulmonary Medical System

As already mentioned, two hundred cases with actual patients' data were used for structuring the Learning Patterns. These were broken up in two parts of 140x60 cases each, as is common practice, in order to build learning and testing samples. This proportion was maintained throughout all the experiments; naturally, cases were randomly selected to take part in a given sample.

The various FFA-ANNs learning terminated when the Medical System could classify properly I/O Patterns up to 100% of correct classification. The numerical convergence error was defined to be 1%, or less. The outcome of the Medical System throughout all the experiments was between 88% and 95%. The present working MDSS has been readjusted to treat all cases correctly.

Tables 3.2 - 3.4 depict the number of Neurons and Synapses of the medical decision support system. The numbers given are overall small in both quantity and magnitude if compared with those of similar applications - thanks to the novelties of the proposed new Medical System. Those numbers are about a System with a novel architecture, new form of ANNs' learning, and an integrated (medical) area to cover: pulmonary diseases. It processes a large number of findings, achieves high speed and operation accuracy and it constitutes the successful product of different collaborating teams of specialists.

Yet, due to a fashion, medical experience is processed and provided - further use of the Medical System is held back mostly due to the use of non-widely accepted Patterns. The understanding and transfer of the acquired knowledge constituted the main aim during the development of the MDSS and the standardization of the medical experience in more generally acceptable rules [H&W90], [E95].

In conclusion, this novel MDSS ensures friendliness, clarity of use, and effectiveness. The first feature is provided by its integration with the CDDM; the second point has already been analysed [§3.8.2]; the third is the product of the harmonic collaboration of many specialists' teams.

	Input	Hidden	Output	Neurons	Synapses
ANN#1	036	015	013	064	0735
ANN#2	016	008	013	037	0232
ANN#3	011	007	013	031	0168
ANN#4	008	004	013	025	0084
ANN#5	004	002	013	019	0034
ANN#6	015	007	013	035	0196
ANN#7	009	005	013	027	0110
ANN#8	013	006	013	032	0156
ANN#9	030	012	013	055	0516
ANN#10	026	002	013	041	0078
ANN#11	026	002	013	041	0078
ANN#12	026	002	013	041	0078
ANN#13	026	002	013	041	0078
ANN#14	026	002	013	041	0078
ANN#15	026	002	013	041	0078
ANN#16	026	002	013	041	0078
ANN#17	026	002	013	041	0078
ANN#18	104	047	013	164	5499
ANN#19	013	000	015	028	0195
Sum	467	129	249	845	8'549

Table 3.2: Neurons and Synapses of Layer #1

	Input	Hidden	Output	Neurons	Synapses
ANN#1	0049	020	035	0104	001680
ANN#2	0029	012	035	0076	000768
ANN#3	0024	010	035	0069	000590
ANN#4	0021	009	035	0065	000504
ANN#5	0017	008	035	0060	000416
ANN#6	0028	011	035	0074	000693
ANN#7	0022	009	035	0066	000513
ANN#8	0026	010	035	0071	000610
ANN#9	0043	018	035	0096	001404
ANN#10	0070	002	035	0107	000210

ANN#11	0070	002	035	0107	000210
ANN#12	0070	002	035	0107	000210
ANN#13	0070	002	035	0107	000210
ANN#14	0070	002	035	0107	000210
ANN#15	0070	002	035	0107	000210
ANN#16	0070	002	035	0107	000210
ANN#17	0070	002	035	0107	000210
ANN#18	0560	283	035	0878	168385
ANN#19	035	000	015	0050	000525
Sum	1'414	406	645	2'465	177'768

Table 3.3: Neurons and Synapses of Layer #2

	Input	Hidden	Output	Neurons	Synapses
ANN #1	0051	021	035	0107	001806
ANN #2	0031	014	035	0080	000924
ANN #3	0026	010	035	0071	000610
ANN #4	0023	009	035	0067	000522
ANN #5	0019	008	035	0062	000432
ANN #6	0030	012	035	0077	000780
ANN #7	0024	009	035	0068	000531
ANN #8	0028	012	035	0075	000756
ANN #9	0045	020	035	0100	001600
ANN#10	0070	002	035	0107	000210
ANN#11	0070	002	035	0107	000210
ANN#12	0070	002	035	0107	000210
ANN#13	0070	002	035	0107	000210
ANN#14	0070	002	035	0107	000210
ANN#15	0070	002	035	0107	000210
ANN#16	0070	002	035	0107	000210
ANN#17	0070	002	035	0107	000210
ANN#18	0560	283	035	0878	168385
ANN #19	015	000	005	0020	000075
Sum	1'412	414	635	2'461	178'101

Table 3.4: Neurons and Synapses of Layer #3 (per set)

3.9 Application of the Medical System in Haematology
The field of pulmonary diseases was chosen as a stepping stone for the application of this Medical System. It was later applied to the field of haematology in order to confirm the research results obtained - also because this field presents some rare features.

It was decided to handle the medical experience gathering with the same methodology and strategy as before - at least in the beginning. As haematology diagnoses also follow the CDDM, no hindrances were expected. However, the morphologic observations of the various medical teams intensify the problem of the developing an appropriate interface between human and machine.

A few differences concerning the **different sizes** of input, output, and hidden Neurons were identified. These are characteristically smaller than those in a MDSS applied to pulmonary diseases [§3.9.1]. The procedure that was followed in integrating the haematology MDSS (H-MDSS) did not vary a lot from the one already described, and thus is not described further.

Moreover, it was necessary to tackle differently the **evaluation** of medical data and laboratory examinations (important in the field of haematology [§3.9.1]), as well as the **displaying** of the results on computer screen. This was somehow expected, as each person perceives differently factors such as: effectiveness, ergonomics, and aesthetics.

The **appearance**, or not, of specialist-considered data as useless (i.e. diseases with small rates of appropriateness) and the way by which findings were **input** changed too. The second team of specialists believe that a Medical System should insulate the non-dominant diseases, examinations, or medical categories.

3.9.1 Grouping of Haematology Medical Data
There were no changes in the core of the Medical System (Patterns processing, medical data's distinctive weights, feeding of data). Specialized MDs of the Haematology Department of the Regional University Hospital of Patras set the specifications, which are referred to the following medical data and findings:
- Pruritus, 10 findings.
- Haemorrhage Manifestations, 8 findings.
- Anaemia, 8 findings.
- Lymphadenopathy, 8 findings.
- Fever, 7 findings.
- Venal Thrombosis, 6 findings.
- Loss of Weight, 5 findings.
- Arterial Embolism, 5 findings.
- Night Sweating, 5 findings.
- Sight Disorders, 3 findings.
- Splenomegaly, 3 findings.
- Leucopenia, 3 findings.

Hence, historic data were again gathered. They were used on the H-MDSS with some differentiations that mainly related to: the smaller number of findings; increase of medical data (due to this fields' nature: blood diseases affect many parts of the body); almost total lack of physical examinations (more related to bulges or the texture of the face and skin), larger number of laboratory examinations, as expected);

much more overlaps of medical elements and findings. As a result, the classification of the probable diseases would have to be based on laboratory examinations. Therefore, great importance was given to the choice and evaluation of the appropriate laboratory examinations. As already mentioned, all comparisons between various MDSSs are considered just before inputting these data [§3.8.2].

This element mainly composes the specific distinction when comparing the two developed Medical Systems. As a consequence, this factor alone (i.e. the plethora of laboratory examinations) probably obstructed the H-MDSS learning.

3.9.2 Architecture of the Haematology Medical System

Fig. 3.1 of this Chapter fully applies again, so Layer #1 of the H-MDSS also responds with appropriateness rates relating to 11 categories of haematology diseases and resultant laboratory examinations. It is also composed by 4 Levels of FFA-ANNs, of three (3) Slabs each, that are connected, as already discussed. The choice of the above units permits the comparison of the two Medical Systems by means of a common study and evaluation base [E94 III, IV].

Layer #2 of the H-MDSS provide as output 25 haematology diseases and the corresponding laboratory examinations. It accepts the outputs of Layer #1 and outputs haematology diseases classification and proposed laboratory examinations.

Layer #3's learning varies much compared to the corresponding of the previous application, since the results of the laboratory examinations were highlighted.

3.9.3 Control and Exploitation of the Haematology Medical System

150 actual patient cases were used this time. They were divided in parts of 100 and 50 cases each and they were utilised by means of experiments organised as before. The accuracy rate of the H-MDSS diagnosis ranged between 83% - 89%, somewhat less than that corresponding to the pulmonary application. This was expected as the laboratory examinations dominate on this application field.

3.10 Conclusions from Exploiting the Two Medical Systems

After the implementation of the H-MDSS too, some early conclusions can be gathered. First, these Medical Systems have not been extensively used. Each one will be characterized mainly during its **operation** in the application field and by the difficulties that will present proper learning and use from/to unskilled MDs.

What is more, they both have been taught with Learning Patterns that were gathered by analysing actual **local** patient cases. The research team will direct their learning towards files of other Greek or international hospitals as some differences might be expected; on the other hand, human experience becomes confined more by the passing of time and the continuous occupation with specialized subjects.

Second, these conclusions have to also consider a number of other factors. As a result, it must not be **falsely considered** that the presented architecture can be applied without problems in all medical fields. The particularity and the mass of data that need processing constitute the most important factors. The accumulated experience of the specialist teams was large and helped to carry the whole project out.

The **development-base**, ensured by the integrated CDDM, appears to be powerful indeed. Essentially, the appropriate control and learning mechanisms are supported and verified continually by an MD. Alternatively, the **adaptability and extensibility** of the novel Medical System constitute a fact. In so much different medical fields of application, a change to the Learning Patterns was sufficient to make a general architecture to stand by itself with similar accuracy.

For the novel Medical Systems, the next targets have been set and some of their elements will be discussed in next chapters, like the improvement of **learning algorithms** [§4.6|7|8], the use of new **ANNs' architectures**, and the utilization of ANNs that will also **process medical images**. Of great interest are also combinations of MDSSs that will handle organs that affect each other (i.e. bronchi-lungs).

3.11 Specialized Utilization of the Novel Medical System

The main target of the research effort in all the duration of the medical decision support system development was its orientation towards applications that would exploit and evolve it in **conditions of every day use**. Its initial application to the fields of pulmonary diseases and haematology proved its great inductive and generalization abilities in the field of medicine and in the development of Medical Systems.

With the extended use of the new Medical System, the necessary requirements are ensured so the **know-how transfer** can be concluded with regards to both the MDSS's implementation and its feeding with new data. As far as its evolution is concerned, more will be discussed in Chapter 8; yet, new specifications concerning its operability will be proposed throughout its use. Its mapping to other areas of human experience will contribute even more to its advancement.

Moreover, the **training** of new pulmonologists and haematologists is facilitated using the Medical System as a teaching tool. In this regard, it could be useful as the appropriate environment for the **confirmation** of symptoms' severity, disease's existence, and treatment aptness, based on actual and imaginary cases, as taken from medical files. The outcome of **corresponding symptoms** when diseases are inputted, constitutes another interesting use. Especially in the case of novel and non-specialized MDs of any field, this choice **resolves** overlapping/fuzzy segments of experience. In addition, the clarity of a diagnosis flow provides the necessary **backing-up argumentation** when deciding on little known diseases.

Finally, an environment was implemented for a **quick, first estimation** of a medical case (although other fields are not excluded). Usually, any time gain importantly reflects on the patient's health and on the conserving of resources, especially in faraway areas, where some specialized tools are not supplied.

The above ideas are only indicative and do not constitute limiting factors for the proper exploitation of the proposed medical decision support system.

3.12 Conclusion

The development and the evolution of a medical decision support system on the fields of pulmonology and haematology was the object of this chapter. Previous Systems mapped in medicine were also studied and their main characteristics were presented. Hence, the principles for the evolution of these "old" Systems have been established and followed, being based on their advantages and disadvantages.

The need to use some specific structures that would cover the demands of specialists who will handle the Medical System, were defined and well established. Through these, the utilization of artificial intelligence techniques easily surfaces as it generally builds up the emulation of the productive induction procedure of the human cognition and the non-standardized specialized experience. Especially, the Artificial Neural Networks seem to dominate as implementation units.

The presented Medical System was integrated by means of a specific ANN architecture, the FFA-ANN, after experiments regarding best Network performance. The same holds true for the ANN chosen learning algorithm; the final result is judged very promising. The research effort has shown a large number of novelties as also open paths toward the creation of more powerful Systems.

For the first time the development of a structure of multiple ANNs and not of a large Network with more intermediate layers is attempted on such a great scale. The learning patterns themselves were not subject to pre-processing whereas the final the System remains flexible enough towards future evolution.

The Medical System, beyond its response accuracy, has also to show several other capabilities and unique characteristics, a consequence of the structure with which it was evaluated and the abilities with which it was equipped. More about its research possibilities will be discussed on the following chapters. Apart from its many traits, its generalization is related to its implementation in hardware.

3.13 References

[Gor73]   Gorry, G. A., "Computer-Assisted Clinical Decision-Making", Meth. Inf. Med., vol. 12, pp. 45-51, 1973

[S&P78]   Szolovits, P. and Pauker, S. G., "Categorical and Probabilistic Reasoning in Medical Diagnosis", AI, vol. 12, pp. 115-144, 1978.

[SBF79]   Shortliffe, E. H., Buchanan, B. G., and Feigenbaum, E. A., "Knowledge Engineering for Medical Decision Making: A Review of Computer-Based Clinical Decision Aids", Proc. of the IEEE, vol. 67, pp. 1207-1224, 1979.

[DeG81]   DeGowin, E. L., DeGowin R. L., "Clinical Examination and Differential Diagnosis", Litsa, Athens, 1981.

[B&S84]   Buchanan, B. G. and Shortliffe, E. H., Rule-Based Expert System: The MYCIN Experiments of the Stanford Heuristic Programming Project, Addison-Wesley, Reading, 1984.

[Alt87]   Alty, J. L., "The Limitations of Rule Based Expert Systems", Knowledge-Based Expert Systems in Industry, Kriz, J. (editor), pp. 17-22, Ellis Horwood Limited, Chichester, 1987.

[Lip87]	Lippmann, R. P., "An Introduction to Computing with NN", IEEE ASSP Mag., vol. 5, pp. 4-22, 1987.
[SPS87]	Schwartz, W. B., Patil, R. S., and Szolovits, P., "AI in Medicine: Where do we Stand?", New Eng. J. of Med., vol. 316, pp. 685-688, 1987.
[Dha88]	Dhawan, A. P., "An ES for the Early Detection of Melanoma Using Knowledge-Based Image Analysis", Anal., Quant. Cyt. and Hist., vol. 10, pp. 405-416, 1988.
[Stu88]	Stubbs, D. F., "Neurocomputers", MD Comp., vol. 5(3), pp. 14-24, 1988.
[Kam89]	Kampschöer, G. H. M., Maruyama, K., van de Velde, C. J. H., Sasako, M., Kinoshita, T., and Okabayashi, K., "Computer Analysis in Making Preoperative Decisions: A Rational Approach to Lymph Node Dissection in Gastric Cancer Patients", Br. J. Surg., vol. 76, pp. 905-908, 1989.
[H&W90]	Hart, A. and Wyatt, J., "Evaluating Black-Boxes as Medical Decision Aids: Issues Arising from a Study of NN", Med. Inf., vol. 15, pp. 229-236, 1990.
[J&F90]	Jacob, R. J. K. and Froscher, J. N., "A Software Engineering Methodology for Rule-Based Systems", IEEE Trans. on Knowl. and Data Eng., vol. 2, pp. 173-189, 1990.
[Mul90]	Mulsant, B. H., "A NN as an Approach to Clinical Diagnosis", MD Comp., vol. 7(1), pp. 25-36, 1990.
[Pol91]	Poli, R., Cagnoni, S., Livi, R., Coppini, G., and Valli, G., "An NN Expert System for Diagnosing and Treating Hypertension", IEEE Comp., vol. 24, pp. 64-71, 1991.
[UMS91]	Umbaugh, S. E., Moss, R. H., and Stoecker, W. V., "Applying Artificial Intelligence to the Identification of Váriegated Coloring in Skin Tumors", IEEE Eng. in Med. and Biol., vol. 10, pp. 57-62, 1991.
[Hen92]	Henson-Mack, K., Chen, H. - C., and Wester, D. C., "Integrating Probabilistic and Rule-Based Systems for CDD", Proc. IEEE SOUTHEASTCON '92, Birm., USA, vol. 2, pp. 699-702, 1992.
[OLe92]	O' Leary, T. J., Mikel, U. V., and Becker, R. L., "Computer-Assisted Image Interpretation: Use of a NN to Differentiate Tubular Carcinoma from Sclerosing Adenosis", Mod. Path., vol. 5, pp. 402-405, 1992.
[S&T92]	Scalero, R. S. and Tepedelenlioglu, N., "A Fast New Algorithm for Training Feedforward NN", IEEE Trans. on Sig. Proc., vol. 40, pp. 202-210, 1992.
[Dur93]	Durg, A., Stoecker, W. V., Cookson, J. P., Umbaugh, S. E., and Moss, R. H., "Identification of Variegating Coloring in Skin Tumors: NN vs. Rule-Based Induction Methods", IEEE Eng. in Med. and Biol., vol. 12, pp. 71-98, 1993.
[E94 I]	Economou, G. - P. K., Spiropoulos, K., Economopoulos, N. M., Charokopos, N., Lymberopoulos, D., Spiliopoulou, M.,

Haralambopulu, E., and Goutis, C. E., "Medical Diagnosis and Artificial Neural Networks: A Medical Expert System applied to Pulmonary Diseases", Proc. of 1994 IEEE NNSP, pp. 482-489, Ermioni, Greece, Sep. 1994.

[E94 II] Economou, G. - P. K., Spiropoulos, K., Economopoulos, N. M., Charokopos, N., Lymberopoulos, D., Spiliopoulou, M., Haralambopulu, E., and Goutis, C. E., "Medical Decision Making Systems in Pulmonology: A Creative Environment based on Artificial Neural Networks", Proc. of 1994 IEEE SMC, pp. 975-980, San Antonio, USA, Oct. 1994.

[E94 III] Economou, G. - P. K., Spiropoulos, K., Economopoulos, N. M., Charokopos, N., Zikos, P., Lymberopoulos, D., and Goutis, C. E., "Decision Supporting Systems in Medical Diseases' Diagnosis: An Artificial Neural Networks Approach", Proc. of Annual Fall Meeting of the Biomedical Society, pp. 123-129, Tempe, USA, Oct. 1994.

[E94 IV] Economou, G. - P. K., Economopoulos, N. M., Charokopos, N., Zikos, P., Lymberopoulos, D., Spiropoulos, K., and Goutis, C. E., "Suggesting Diagnosis of Diseases and Treatment: How far Artificial Neural Networks can go?", Proc. of 1994 IEEE ISANN, pp. 626-631, Tainan, Taiwan, Dec. 1994.

[E95] Economou, G. - P. K., Economopoulos, N. M., Lymberopoulos, D., and C. E. Goutis, "Experiences Accumulated Working towards Medical Decision Support Systems", J. of Microprocessing and Microprogramming, vol. 40, pp. 883-886, 1995.

4th Chapter

Artificial Neural Network Learning Procedure

Just as electricity knows its conductor,
or vacuum knows its limit...
R. Zelazny

4.1 Introduction

Artificial Neural Networks' development is mainly focused on their Learning Algorithms. The already-proposed and well-exploited Artificial Neurons and the ANNs' architectures constitute model structures (mainly because of their acceptable imitation of their biological analogues) and demonstrate good performances. So far no new ideas have been put forward to establish new propositions. Moreover, researchers orientate their algorithms towards obtaining ANNs' certain convergence into Learning Patterns and less towards their faster execution.

Only during the last years research has taken a firm interest on the last issue, despite this being the slowest stage of the ANNs' use. It takes place only few times on an application Network, before its final set-up; later on its superior processing speed and response accuracy have the first word. Moreover, the development in electronic circuits integration technology (VLSI chips) has been a contributing factor in increasing the processing speed.

Gradually, the on-chip learning grew into a necessity, independently from the ANNs' architecture [S&C91, C&T94, H&P94]. Also, with the use of integrated circuits some space and building restrictions were exceeded (many Neurons can be implemented on a chip - both digital or analogue ones) and the need for further developing those algorithms emphasized on their application speed [MMC94]. Few of them though, can be implemented on silicon without serious changes.

Moreover, the ANNs' convergence into the available Learning Patterns, as a methodology, is conditioned by much ambiguity [§1.3]. Defining only the known parameters of Networks (architecture, number, and type of Neurons, etc.) does not complete the subdivision procedure of the Reference Space in the Classes where the Patterns belong. The different emphasis of each resulting sub-space and the right balance between them require a different analysis [§1.3].

Finally, the creation, the learning, and the adaptation of ANNs in this book's applications, is primarily related to the successive approximation of the FFA-ANN's size (number of hidden Slabs/Neurons [§1.2]). Methodologies are therein described that were tested in-the-field and their results are analyzed and explained under a new estimation and research topic - the one concerning Weights.

4.2 Forms of Learning Patterns

It is a common belief that the largest section of human brain, approximately 80%, remains "unused". The assumption laying behind such a simple estimation, is related to the referenced period of time. The researched scientific beliefs state that the whole brain is used but during the mind's learning process.

The "unused" part of the brain cells (biological neurons) can be characterized as such, only when it is considered that the biological synapses are finally set. Besides, the whole learning procedure and how this is related to the brain activity, is still unknown territory. The newest considerations correlate the huge mass of brain cells with the intellect, as a necessary action for human learning, regardless of the partial connecting "schemes" of the biological neurons when they form biological neural networks. Because of this fact, human beings learn more easily at a young age, when the "unused" neurons have yet to start decreasing in numbers. In direct association, redundant Neurons are also present in ANNs (in their hidden Slabs), after they "learn" (converge into their Learning Patterns).

The exploitation of Weights in this book as a means to have better Learning Algorithms, will concentrate in the FFA-ANN as it constitutes the most common Network - the most recent applications are based on it. A Network's learning quality and demands, and its convergence depend on the use of the correct number of Neurons in its hidden Slab and of the Learning Patterns' and Learning Algorithm form. The term "learning quality" indicates whether the Network's convergence results in **memorization** or **correlation** of the Patterns [§1.3].

The Patterns' correlation denotes the creation of logical connections between them and the number of hidden Neurons that will be demanded during the ANNs' Learning. On occasions, it is even achieved without the insertion of specific Patterns in a Network (the specialist ignored some of the correlations [Pol91]). "Many" Neurons generally ensure faster convergence (compare with biological ones) but they also might lead into a non-correlation. The memorization, a non-correlation (final) situation, characterizes an ANN's learning in which semantic Pattern association was not created, thus reminding the human "parrot learning".

With the memorization, an ANN is degenerated to function as a look-up table or data storage memory, into which new (unknown) inputs, corrupted, or/and incomplete input patterns of the ones already memorized, are generally fed. The Network outputs should then constitute the learnt forms of those inputs (output Patterns), consequently actualizing a "noise" extraction from the fed inputs.

As far as **convergence** of the input Learning Patterns to the output ones is concerned, the hidden Neurons may simply not be enough [Lip87] as it will be shown next. On the other hand, the **demands** of a Network in electronic data indicate its necessary Neurons for its probable mapping in hardware or software.

The internationally accepted policy for inputting Learning Patterns in an ANN takes place as an **one to one** and **on to mapping** of input to output Patterns elements (vectors). Generally, pairs of input and output vectors are fed to the Network (separately or in sets of distinguished pairs); the initially random set 'Weights' weigh the inputs; the ANN's outputs fire; its difference from the wanted value is calculated (output error); and this value is then propagated backwards in order to readjust the Weights by means of a Learning Algorithm [§1.2].

This learning scheme takes for granted the **mapping** and **representation** capability of the input data into unambiguous Learning Patterns that must not turn out in successively devaluating them. This problem is faced mostly by increasing the input vectors' components or by feeding the ANN with more Patterns.

The existence of a **"capable" number** of input/output data - that will form the Learning Patterns, and where it is possible, the assurance that they cover the related space - constitutes another assumption. The Patterns should form the outcome of an appropriate process and be independent, without overlapping areas.

Finally, the ANN's development should ensure the modulation of the Network's space into sub-fields (classes) [§1.2] without the developer's **intervention**, in order to exclude any external (to the application) leading factors beyond the Learning Algorithm itself. The ANNs treated in this book converged by means of Algorithms taken from the bibliography and as far as Medical Systems are considered, their functionality was extensively tested by MDs by means of many unknown inputs [§3.8.3, §3.9.3].

The above input to output vectors mapping is characterized as an **output-centred ("Form-1")** learning. In other words, it is considered important for an ANN to converge in a (stable) condition where each output vector component will be triggered separately from the others. The input vectors on the other hand, are composed by elements whose position and relations are as defined by the application. Despite its common practice form, it also has many disadvantages.

The need for supplying **clearly defined** input sets, that shall promote an output component each, is one. It demands input vectors formed by elements with a very low to inexistent uncertainty percentage in their every value.

The difficulty to separately assign a distinctive **importance** to each separate element of the input vectors, as the development of the integral vector comes first, impedes the classification of data by means of their single characteristics. Also, **weakness** to assign a set of inputs to more than one output, forces the ANN into non-accepting the overlapping medical symptomatology as learning data.

Fig. 4.1 shows the "Form-1" for a pair of Patterns. The eight (8) elements of the input vector trigger only one (1) of the output elements in the logical "1".

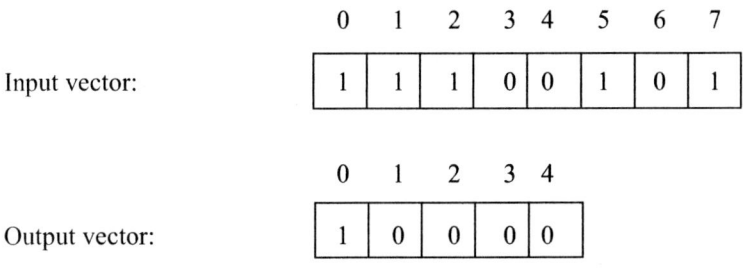

Figure 4.1: Learning Patterns "Form-1" Input and Output Vectors

In the above figure, the logical "1" represents a vector's element existence, whereas the logical "0" a vector's element non-existence. The suspicion about or the indifference in a vector's element value is not represented [E94, E95 I].

4.3 The Output-centred Learning Patterns' Form

In the evolutionary course of our search towards a (medical) decision support system, the Learning Patterns' "Form-1" was used first. The aforementioned disadvantages and the next ones were observed so that a new form of Patterns was proposed and fully utilized. To better understand it, let us suppose that an FFA-ANN was to be trained by means of the following Patterns (Fig. 4.2):

	0	1	2	3	4	5	6	7
Input vector 1:	1	1	1	0	0	1	0	1
Input vector 2:	1	1	1	1	0	0	0	1
Input vector 3:	1	1	1	1	0	1	?	?

Figure 4.2: Three Contrasted Learning Patterns "Form-1" Input Vectors

First feature to observe is that the first two (2) vectors **differ little** (in their third and fifth component). Therefore, if the first is fed as a new (unknown) input to an ANN (i.e. after its learning), then the corresponding (to this vector) output will be triggered up to a 100% of its logical "1's" physical mapping (its actual hardware or software value), whereas the same output would be triggered up to a 80% of its logical "1" (relative resemblance) should the second vector also be fed to the said ANN. In addition, the corresponding to this input (vector 2) output will also be triggered up to a 100% of its logical "1's" physical mapping. That could well constitute, at the specialized MD or/and expert's opinion, error and disorientation of outcomes, as they might prefer a non-triggered output at all.

The second point to take into consideration concerns the **integrity** of Patterns. If the third vector is fed to the ANN, and the "?" element is mapped as a logical "0.5", then the corresponding to the first and second vectors outputs will both be triggered up to a 62.5%% of their logical "1's" physical mapping (relative resemblance, again). To solve this misfit, special values could be given to some of the vectors' elements [§3.8.1] (now non effective). Those elements should be more strictly set and not be "counted" only for their presence but also for their particular place in the vector.

The third point to be observed also concerns the third vector. It constitutes the most common form of input (be it a Pattern or unknown one), since seldom the medical (or other) data are **inserted in their full form**. Usually, less important elements are skipped, although they have to be considered as inputs during the learning due to the cognition their existence or not may inherit to the ANN [§3.8.1, §3.9.1]. The uncertainty's representation should then be standardized.

As a result, the need arises to build a new structure of input/output vectors to form Learning Patterns. They could also be fragmented, depending on their value, and separately fed in ANNs; or else the use of several Networks with overlapping roles that would handle more or less basic Patterns, could be another solution. However, the later one is rejected, as experimental results convinced us that such an implementation would not bring the outcome to fruition.

Besides, this latter solution does **not add safety** in an ANN's output. In medicine, and by extension in many areas of human experience, there "are no diseases but patients". Likewise, there are no "main" Patterns but incident cases that both specialized MDs and Medical Systems ought to uniformly examine. A possible Patterns' fragmentation would yield input data's degeneration.

Moreover, fragmentation would require **excessive time** for gathering and reallocating data and would mean the adaptation of the specialists (i.e. the MDs) on the experience field, as they are not taught with under this logic. Yet, this data reallocation constitutes an element of their experience (induction); i.e. can be only explained by means of more Patterns than those they can describe. In total, it can be said that is **non-practical** and **foreign** to the utilization of ANNs, as in this manner their feature to correlate input data would not be properly exploited.

4.4 The Proposed Input-centred Learning Patterns' Form

In this section, the reversal of the Learning Patterns' form is proposed, from output-centred to a new, **input-centred** mapping ("**Form-2**"). The reasons that led to it are summarized in the need for bestowing enhanced factors **performance** in the input vector's elements. Also, its importance is to be sought in the previous chapter analysis [§3.8.1]. Moreover, the **ineffectiveness** of "Form-1" to describe the special importance between each findings per disease backs up this choice.

Another reason is the **asymmetry** in the subdivision of the reference space (medicine) in classes (categories of- and diseases) by means of using the "Form-1" [§1.3]. Input Patterns with fewer elements underwent better resemblance rates to their respective outputs (during the insertion of new inputs) than those that were displaying more elements during learning (due to their larger chance of having more elements present in the new input vector). As it has already been mentioned, the feeding of findings in "Form-1" by means of Patterns segregation rather deteriorated, than enhanced, the Medical System's performance.

Following the proposed "Form-2" mapping, each input element is separately fed into the Network. These are three logical data levels defined as follows [§3.8.1]:

- The **logical "1"**, wherever present in a "Form-1" input vector, is used to separately form a single input vector of the same number of elements as the one it came from; it keeps its place and each of rest elements of the vector (i.e. findings of a symptom), is set to the **logical "0.5"** (do not care element).
- The number of "Form-1" elements set to the logical "1" value is kept **constant** and equal to the largest number of logical "1"s input elements of all outputs, for all "Form-2" input vectors (normalization). Should there be "Form-1" input vectors lacking in logical "1"s, **pseudo-inputs** are inserted in "Form-2" input vectors. Those could constitute future medicine findings (per disease).

- A "Form-2" input vector is **correlated** to an output one whose each element is set to the logical "1" according to its triggering or not by the input element.
- **Weight factors** can be given to each separate input element (finding).
- The **logical "0"** is indirectly used since an output element is triggered by only a given input one. The lack of inputs does not trigger any output.
- A Pattern full of only **logical "0.5"**'s is also fed to the ANN. Its existence is for triggering all the outputs, something that is explained from a System's point of view (inputs' balance), medicine (when in ambiguity, promote all the outputs), and the operating flow of intermediate decisions by the System (lack of data promotes all the outputs that will be made clear by means of laboratory examinations).

The following section's example explains, describes, and makes clear the mapping steps towards "Form-2" Learning Patterns' input/output vectors.

4.5 Application of the "Form-2" of the Learning Patterns
Let us have the following input vectors, of four elements each, and their corresponding outputs, as they are described in the next figure (Fig. 4.3).

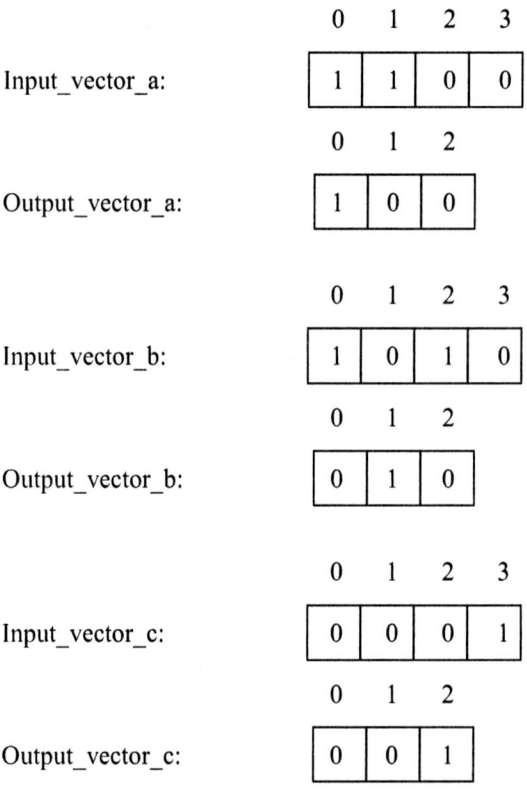

Figure 4.3: Learning Patterns "Form-1" I/O Vectors

The "Form-1" input_vector_a has two logical "1"s; therefore, it will have to form two "Form-2" different input vectors. As a result, during the first transformation step, it will be made as follows (Fig. 4.4):

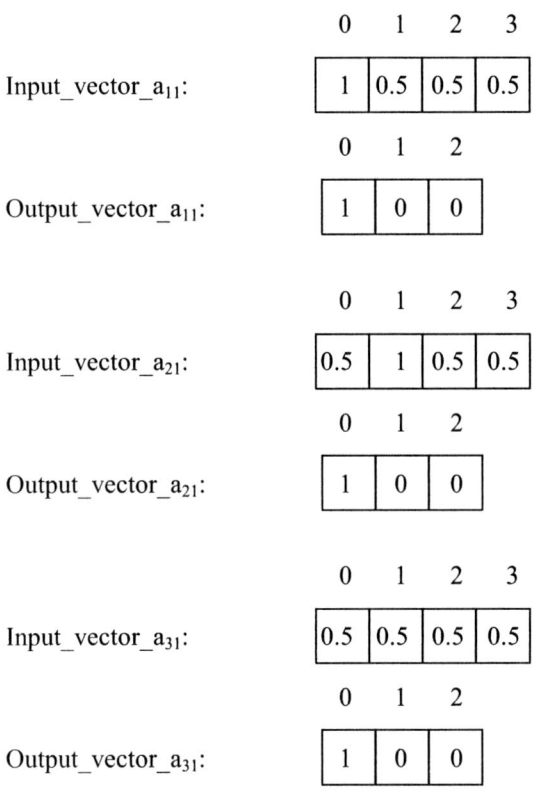

Figure 4.4: Transformed input_vector_a (intermediate_form_1)

"Form-2" input_vector_a_{11} is a result of the logical "1" that "Form-1" input_vector_a has in its 0th position. The same holds true for "Form-2" input_vector_a_{12} that is a result of the logical "1" that "Form-1" input_vector_a has in its 1st position. However, "Form-2" input_vector_a_{31} is a biased input.

On the other hand, "Form-2" output_vector_a_{11}, output_vector_a_{21}, and output_vector_a_{31}, are identical to "Form-1" output_vector_a, as expected.

The "Form-1" input_vector_b also has two logical "1"s; therefore, it will have to form two "Form-2" different input vectors. As a result, during the first transformation step, it will be made as follows (Fig. 4.5):

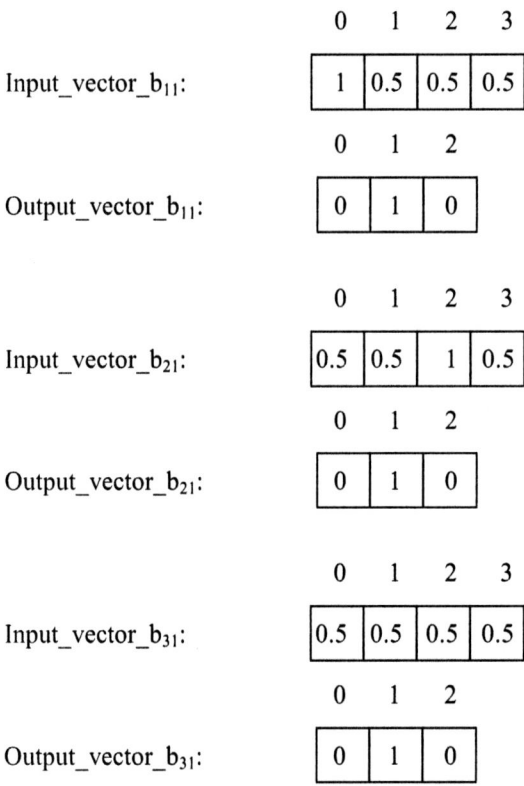

Figure 4.5: Transformed input_vector_b (intermediate_form_1)

"Form-2" input_vector_b_{11} is a result of the logical "1" that "Form-1" input_vector_b has in its 0th position. The same holds true for "Form-2" input_vector_b_{12} that is a result of the logical "1" that "Form-1" input_vector_b has in its 3d position. However, "Form-2" input_vector_b_{31} is a biased input. The reader can see that "Form-2" input_vector_a_{11} and input_vector_b_{11} are identical and are correlated to different outputs ("Form-2" output_vector_a_{11} and output_vector_b_{11}), a fact that "Form-1" could have handled properly. The same holds true (again) for "Form-2" input_vector_a_{31} and input_vector_b_{31}.

On the other hand, "Form-2" output_vector_b_{11}, output_vector_b_{21}, and output_vector_b_{31}, are identical to "Form-1" output_vector_b, as expected.

The "Form-1" input_vector_c has only one logical "1"; therefore, it will have to form one "Form-2" input vector as well. As a result, during the first transformation step, it will be made as follows (Fig. 4.6):

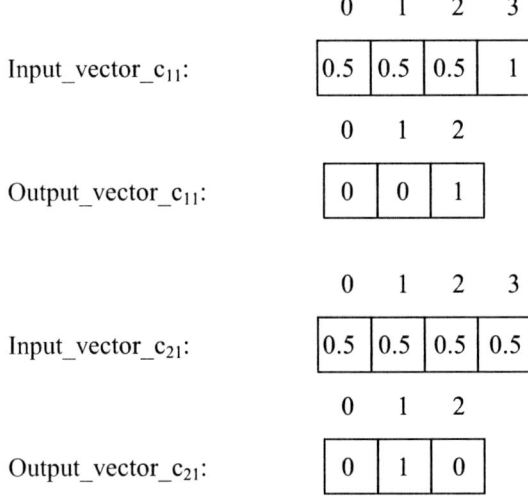

Figure 4.6: Transformed input_vector_c (intermediate_form_1)

"Form-2" input_vector_c_{11} is a result of the logical "1" that "Form-1" input_vector_c has in its 3d position. However, "Form-2" input_vector_c_{21} is a biased input. The reader can see that "Form-2" input_vector_a_{31}, input_vector_b_{31}, and input_vector_c_{21}, are identical and are correlated to different outputs ("Form-2" output_vector_a_{31}, output_vector_b_{31}, and output_vector_c_{21}).

On the other hand, "Form-2" output_vector_c_{11} and output_vector_c_{21} are identical to "Form-1" output_vector_c, as expected.

Despite all itermediate_form_1 conversions from "Form-1' to "Form-2" I/O Learning Patterns, the above transformations do not constitute the final mapping of inputs and outputs vectors of "Form-2". That is because the maximum number of logical "1"s in "Form-1" representation is two for any given output, therefore each input vector will have to form two "Form-2" ones. Consequently, input_vector_c will have to be given an additional (pseudo-)input.

Therefore, in order to complete the normalization of input components correctly [§1.3, §4.4], the Patterns shown in the next figures are created (Fig. 4.7-4.9). Yet, the reader is reminded that pseudo-inputs are only utilized to form Learning Patterns. During the supply of new (unknown) inputs in FFA-ANNs, pseudo-inputs are nor fed neither appear during the performance control of the Networks [3.8.3, 3.9.3]. However, they do participate in the Weights' evaluation.

Since "Form-1" input_vector_a has two logical "1"s, its intermediate_form_2 I/O vectors will be identical to its intermediate_form_1 ones with the addition of a do not care pseudo-input (to the input vectors). As a result, during the second transformation step, they will be made as follows (Fig. 4.7):

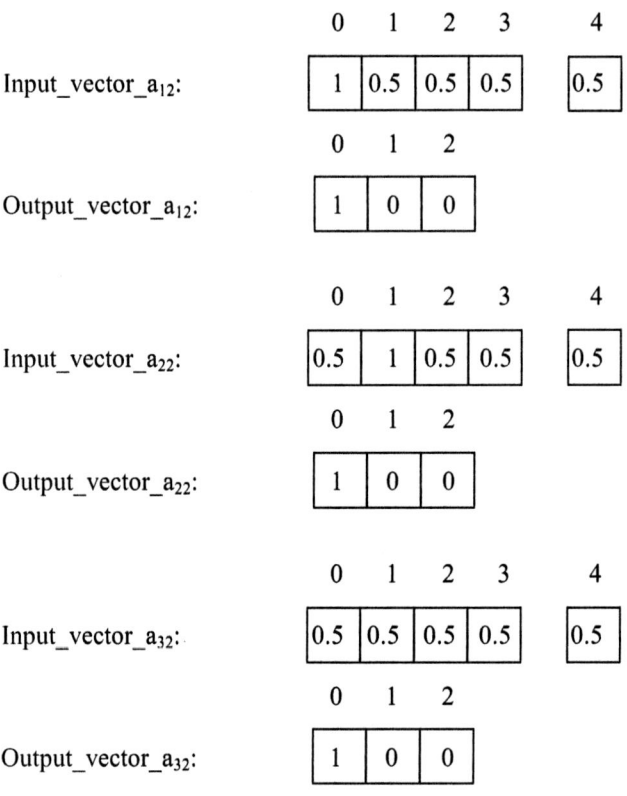

Figure 4.7: Transformed input_vector_a (intermediate_form_2)

"Form-2" input_vector_a_{12} is a result of the logical "1" that "Form-1" input_vector_a has in its 0th position and an added do not care pseudo-input. The same holds true for "Form-2" input_vector_a_{22} that is a result of the logical "1" that "Form-1" input_vector_a has in its 1st position and an added do not care pseudo-input. "Form-2" input_vector_a_{32} remains a biased input plus the added do not care pseudo-input. Also, "Form-2" output_vector_a_{12}, output_vector_a_{22}, and output_vector_a_{32}, are identical to "Form-1" output_vector_a, as expected.

Since "Form-1" input_vector_b has two logical "1"s, its intermediate_form_2 I/O vectors will be identical to its intermediate_form_1 ones with the addition of a do not care pseudo-input (to the input vectors). As a result, during the second transformation step, they will be made as follows (Fig. 4.8):

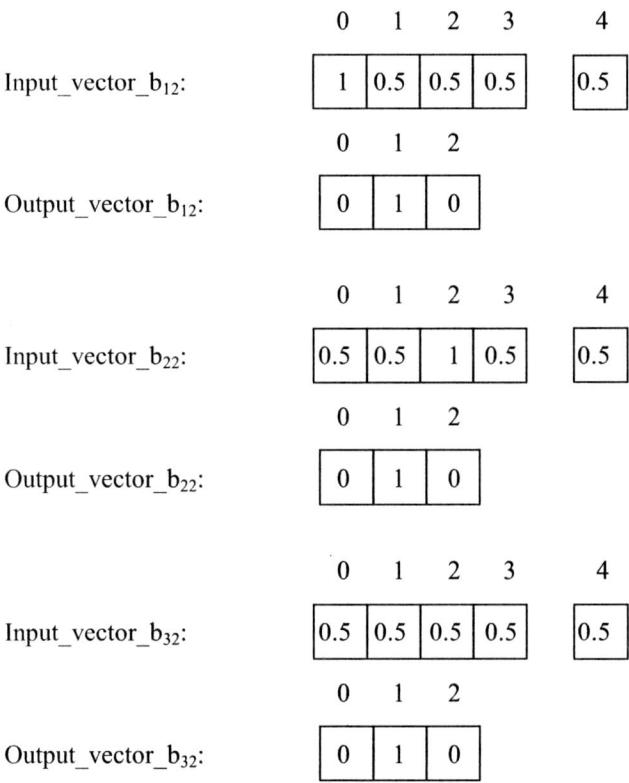

Figure 4.8: Transformed input_vector_b (intermediate_form_2)

"Form-2" input_vector_b_{12} is a result of the logical "1" that "Form-1" input_vector_a has in its 0th position and an added do not care pseudo-input. The same holds true for "Form-2" input_vector_b_{22} that is a result of the logical "1" that "Form-1" input_vector_b has in its 3d position and an added do not care pseudo-input. "Form-2" input_vector_b_{32} remains a biased input plus the added do not care pseudo-input. The reader can see that "Form-2" input_vector_a_{12} and input_vector_b_{12} are identical and are correlated to different outputs ("Form-2" output_vector_a_{12} and output_vector_b_{12}). The same holds true (again) for "Form-2" input_vector_a_{32} and input_vector_b_{32} (as aforementioned).

Also, "Form-2" output_vector_b_{12}, output_vector_b_{22}, and output_vector_b_{32}, are identical to "Form-1" output_vector_b, as expected.

Since "Form-1" input_vector_c has one logical "1"s, its intermediate_form_2 I/O vectors will be identical to its intermediate_form_1 ones with the addition of do not care (to the already transformed input vectors) and an additional input vector with a logical "1" pseudo-input. As a result, during the second transformation step, they will be made as follows (Fig. 4.9):

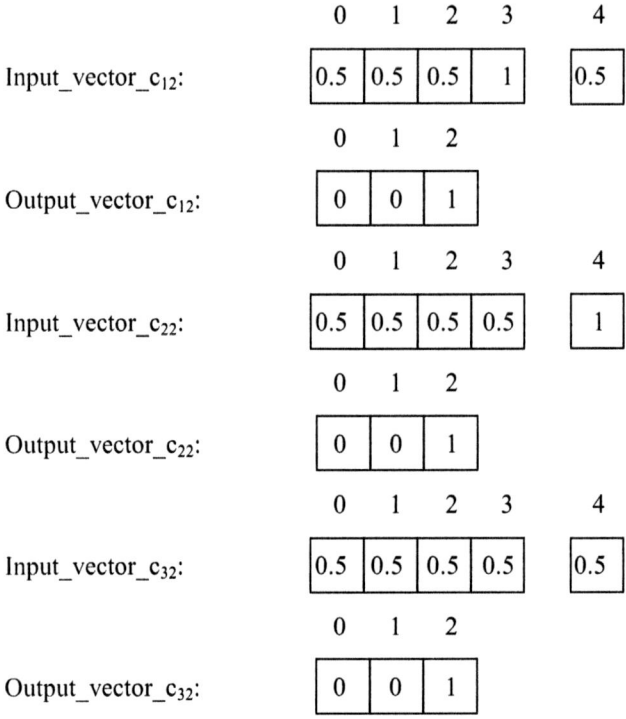

Figure 4.9: Transformed input_vector_c (intermediate_form_2)

"Form-2" input_vector_c_{12} is a result of the logical "1" that "Form-1" input_vector_c has in its 3d position and an added do not care pseudo-input. "Form-2" input_vector_c_{22} is a result of the addition of a logical "1" pseudo-input in order to normalize input vectors (as already explained). "Form-2" input_vector_c_{32} is a biased input plus the added do not care pseudo-input. The reader can see that "Form-2". The reader can see that "Form-2" input_vector_a_{32}, input_vector_b_{32}, and input_vector_c_{32}, are identical and are correlated to different outputs ("Form-2" output_vector_a_{32}, output_vector_b_{32}, and output_vector_c_{32}).

On the other hand, "Form-2" output_vector_c_{12}, output_vector_c_{22}, and output_vector_c_{32} are identical to "Form-1" output_vector_c, as expected.

Finally, the special factors are left to be applied in each logical "1" [§3.8.1] in the "Form-2" intermediate_form_2 elements. Those vary by depending on the specialist's opinion. In medical applications, their classification into four levels was proved to be sufficient (Table 3.1). Their application will not be shown in the presented example (due to the lack of the proper input data); however, they are only "boosting" multiplication percentages. Therefore, the final I/O Learning Pattern vectors with which the FFA-ANN of the example would be taught are modulated as presented on the following figure (Fig. 4.10):

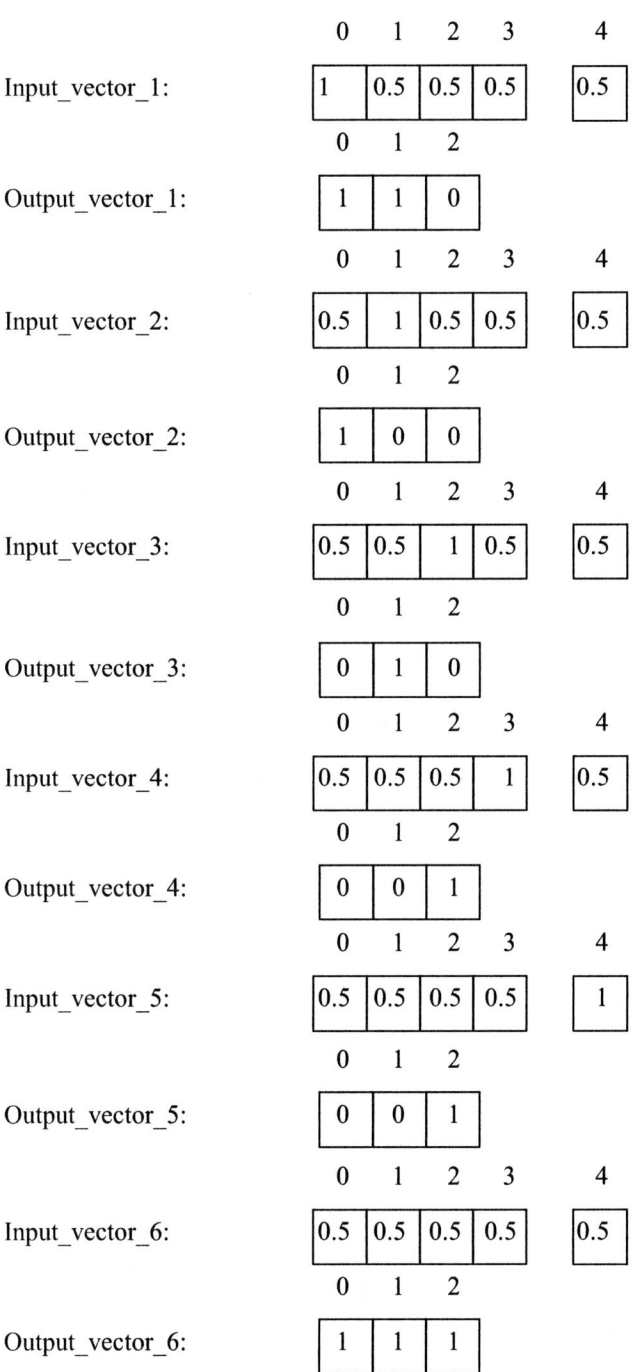

Figure 4.10: Learning Patterns "Form-2" I/O Vectors

The reader can see that "Form-2" input vectors that were previously present (see intermediate_form_1 and intermediate_form_2) and triggered different outputs (see previous figures) are no longer existent. Each complete "Form-2" output vector is now only triggered by a separate, single "Form-2" input vector.

A number of advantages from the structuring the I/O Learning Patterns by means of "Form-2" mapping, follows next. First, there **is no output** that is not "responding", even partially, to each input, because of FFA-ANNs' topology and thanks to the feeding of Learning Patterns that is offered to the Networks. Consequently, even the smallest level of possible existence for a given output class is promoted by the more general decision support system and is either enhanced or degraded on the next stages, or is appropriately faced by the specialized user. Each output responds to different appropriateness levels [§3.7, §3.8.2].

The application of the special factors to each input element has been previously highlighted. Only this Patterns mapping, though, places it **in its correct base**, as in each input component a separate value can be given. It constitutes an elegant, adaptable and evolvable method of values representation.

Moreover, FFA-ANNs are responding now even to **incomplete findings**, as the non existent elements in input vectors can be utilized; moreover that fact inducts a different logic use and combination of their results (i.e. should in an new input vector be used as existent or not), depending on the judgment and experience of the specialist who provides his/her knowledge.

The **number** of the outcome inputs and outputs is calculated before the mapping to the "Form-2" of the Patterns' components. At the same time, the appearance of **partial Patterns and inputs** is not anymore a cause for their definitive rejection, as the System's respond is based on the separately enhanced special characteristics, that the rest of an input vector's elements present.

4.6 Assessment of the Hidden Neurons

The hidden Neurons define the storage of Learning Patterns in FFA-ANNs by means of the Synapses that connect them to the Network's inputs and outputs [Lip87, T&P89]. Despite the fact that those Networks are applied in a large scale, few elements have been clarified with regards to hidden Neurons' important functioning as the mechanisms that govern it concern a huge number of Synapses. The number of the hidden Slabs and Neurons, their characteristics and their connecting schemes with the rest of the Slabs (full or partial), constitute a subject of extensive research. In addition, ANNs' applications are characterized by considerable variety, leading the appliance of metrical or statistic rules to fail.

Some of the hidden Slabs qualities can be exploited, e.g. it only takes **three** of them, at most, for a Network to converge at an adequate error threshold [Lip87]. Also, hidden Neurons' numbers are usually defined on an **experimental** basis:

- due to their **correlation** to distinguished categories. $v(2v + 1)$ hidden Neurons are sufficient for the classification of a given space to v sub-fields (classes) [Lip87].

- following a **maximum upper limit** scheme. Mirchandani and Cao [M&C89] state that κ Neurons suffice for the linear differentiation of Y sub-fields at most in a δ-dimensional field, while

$$Y(\kappa, \delta) = \sum_{i=0}^{\delta} \binom{\kappa}{i}, \left[\binom{\kappa}{i} = 0, \kappa < i\right]$$

- **developing adaptive algorithms** [HYH90] which, depending on the convergence development, alter the number of hidden Neurons.

The assessment of the number of hidden Slabs/Neurons is important in the proper utilization of the Learning Patterns. Researchers' criteria try to find:
- Hidden Slabs/Neurons number.
- Completeness of the reference space account.
- Best convergence accuracy.

Usually, some numbers are chosen and correction takes place afterwards.

The Weights that correspond to the Synapses, present particular **interest** both for their **values'** distribution and for their representation in a graph of Synapses (patterns of "mountains" and "valleys" [§4.7]) that correlate the Neurons' activity (according to their larger/smaller values), and generally their firing performance.

For both MDSSs, the number of Patterns was held in exceptionally low levels [§4.7]. The number of hidden Neurons was defined with the "$v(2v + 1)$" rule, and the "Form-2" mapping permitted the classes' creation in few Learning Cycles.

Experiments conducted in the field of medicine (pulmonary diseases and haematology) proved the sufficiency of only a hidden Slab for the required learning threshold.

When needed, the adding of more hidden Neurons was kept to a low number (one to two), so that **correlation,** and not **memorizing** during the Network's learning, was ensured. A useful step for examining the **qualitative difference** in ANNs' learning, and for the previous "generation" of Weights to be **re-used** [E95 II].

To prove further the last observation, a Network's learning was not restored to its zero base (selection of random values for the Weights), as the back propagation rule defines, in order to start a new Learning Period for an ANN with a plus/minus hidden Neuron than before, but this initialization was applied only in the new Synapses. Old Synapses kept their values. In that way, extra learning time was averted (saved 18%-20% average time), and useful conclusions were reached.

The utilization of the "$v(2v + 1)$" and the **maximum upper limit** rules, for obtaining the hidden Neurons [Lip87, M&C89] constitute a reliable starting base. The **redundancy,** though, of the surplus hidden Neurons number should be conserved until the final convergence is reached, as the classification to groups of more or less active hidden Neurons, is better made. Yet, the removal of the hidden Neurons that seem to "be in excess" and the ANNs' without them re-learning, do not particularly decrease the Network's total topology and it was not further tested.

4.7 The Synapses' Weights

Researchers worldwide usually refer to the ANNs' hidden Slab(s) as the elements that process the inputs (separate the reference space in classes) and feed the output (map the classes into known responses) [T&P89], [§1.2]. Similarly, the Synapses' Weights to and from the hidden Slabs constitute the parameters of those elements.

It has also been observed that some (human, etc.) decisions depend more on specific input elements. Hence, among the Synapses' Weights there can be find some **Weight groups'** participation to a decision (the output's firing "path").

By means of the higher-valued (in absolute terms) Weights, some outputs can be either strengthened or inactivated, thus demonstrating a "decision rule's" lead. This can be exploited by an **expert system** that will be set as a controller of an ANN. Moving towards this direction, algorithms having structures of the type "if... then... else", fuzzy logic systems [L&L91], and rules of linear data regression [T&P89] are developed to formulate those rules, up to a degree.

The latter control techniques can be especially used in combination to decision support systems [§2.4]. However, as the previous analysis has already shown, a number of disadvantages (e.g. harm to the correlation schemes Learning Patterns impart to ANNs) probably accompany such efforts.

A study of the Synapses' Weights can clarify the association among the biologically-simulated phenomenon of Neurons' **firing** and its importance for their function [§1.2]. International bibliography proposes specific models for this analysis by detecting the position of Neurons in ANNs, of their Weights, and the special response in specific inputs [T&P89].

Moreover, such a study clarifies the input Patterns' **quality**: the existence or non-existence of dominant characteristics, the need of utilizing or not normalized Patterns, and the output values' correct threshold classification.

In addition, it could explain the **adequacy or not** of the hidden Neurons, since many very high values of the Weights, that can be incited by the lack of hidden Neurons, may lead an ANN to no further learning, to show weakness in creating correlations between the Patterns, and to make difficult the transition in hardware [§6.4]. Of course, it could also demonstrate the **redundancy** of hidden Neurons. Research for decreasing this redundancy is opposed to the previous analysis about (a good) ANN's convergence, so that a "productive" compromise is sought.

All the above point only to a qualitative tone in specifying the Weights importance because specific interventions in Weights' mode of employment are based on heuristic rules. It must also be noted that an efficiently-operating application is seldom modified, but it is surpassed by future demand; also, as far as changes are concerned they are usually handled before the start an ANN operation's.

A systematic effort for the formulation of general rules that will change Weights during or after the ANNs' convergence, beyond the effects of the Learning Algorithm, is also hindered by the Networks' **application extent**. The ANNs solve problems that differ in application, in their Patterns' representation, in their learning, in their architecture or in their hardware/software implementation, so that a specific correlation of outputs, Weights and Neurons, is not applied in a more general scale. However, intervening in ANNs whose convergence in Patterns led to memorization or to their correlation, would accept only different treatments.

On the other hand, a probable use of **hybrid systems** that are used by ANNs and other artificial intelligence applications does not assist the research. Such systems usually operate better than single applications, but due to their complex structure they do not simply reflect the Networks' traits but probably the overall system's response. A screening of each parts' effect cannot always be achieved.

4.8 Approximations for Less Hardware and Faster Convergence

Mainly heuristic techniques are applied after an FFA-ANNs Learning Period so as to decrease the number of the redundant hidden Neurons [HYH90]. Experimental results (teaching and controlling FFA-ANN's performance) confirmed that:

- **Redundancy** in hidden Neurons number constitutes a disadvantage only in the case of memorized Learning Patterns. It partially augments the ANNs' characteristics and improves their future generalization into unknown inputs by, accordingly, demanding more silicon/memory area. Thus, efforts to decrease memory demand should follow after convergence.

- The hidden Slabs/Neurons that are removed should be chosen so as not to disturb the **balance** on the basis of which the structuring of sub-fields (classes), out of the reference space, was accomplished. The higher-valued (in absolute terms) Weights must be kept (and so are the Neurons linked by them), or preserve their functionality by obtaining re-convergence of the rest of the ANN.

- Before attempting any changes on the Weights' number or values, an analysis of their function must be performed to decrease the **total** convergence time.

Emphasis should be given to the fact that interventions in FFA-ANNs' Weights make sense only for large Networks and while implementing of on-chip Learning Algorithms. The ANN convergence without any interventions, no matter how slow it can be, is achieved as long as the Patterns are properly formed [§4.4].

Conversely, those interventions should not be done by non developers. Some features of artificial neural networks, that have not been explored, ought to be preserved as they may be relate to the Network structure during the convergence (e.g. mapping of Patterns, maximum/minimum Weights' values).

If chip area is required (hardware implementation) and the Weights cannot be changed (in value or number), the problem may also be solved with the appropriate design techniques and the use of external memories [§6.5]. Fig. 4.11-4.22, show the evolution of Weights for the "Cough's" ANN.

As the reader can see, during the Learning Period, variable "valleys" (depressions of the graph) and "hills" (peaks of the graph) are fashioned. Some of those undergo serious re-shaping until the convergence criteria are reached, whereas some others keep their features. Through all the experiments, interventions to alter the Synapses' Weights concluded to [E95 II]:

88

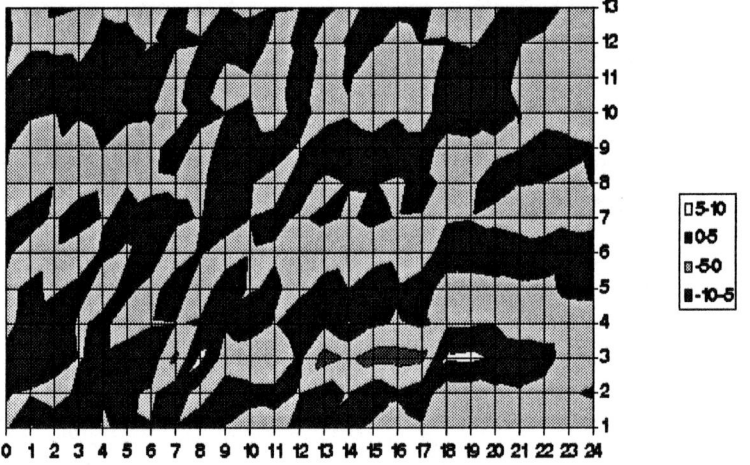

x-axis denote input and y-axis hidden Neurons

Figure 4.11: Synapses' Weights (150th Cycle)

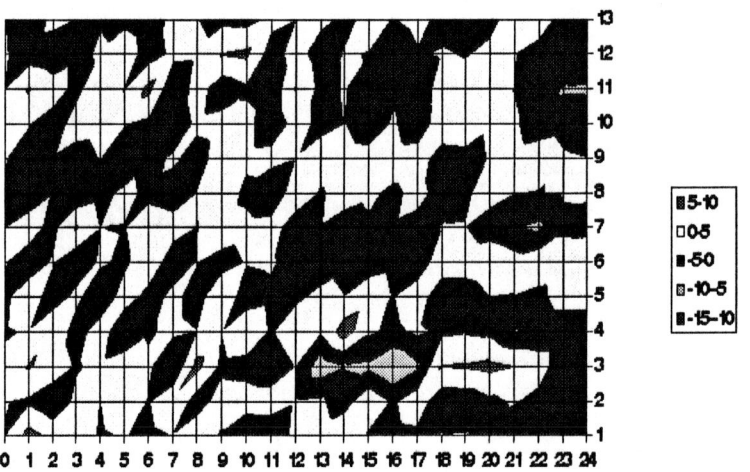

x-axis denote input and y-axis hidden Neurons

Figure 4.12: Synapses' Weights (300th Cycle)

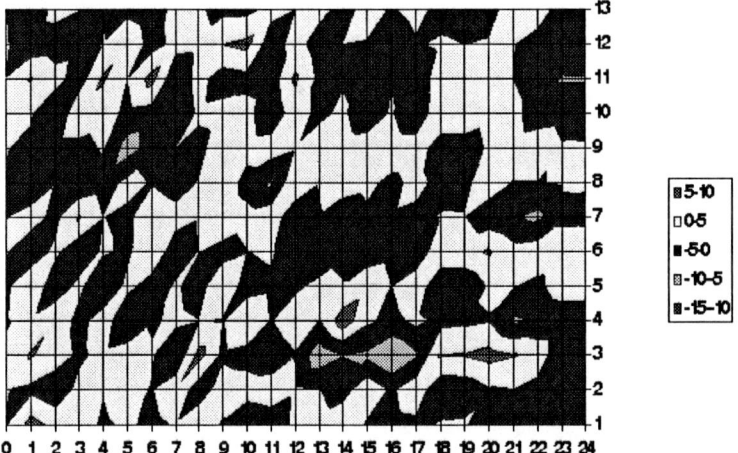

x-axis denote input and y-axis hidden Neurons

Figure 4.13: Synapses' Weights (450th Cycle)

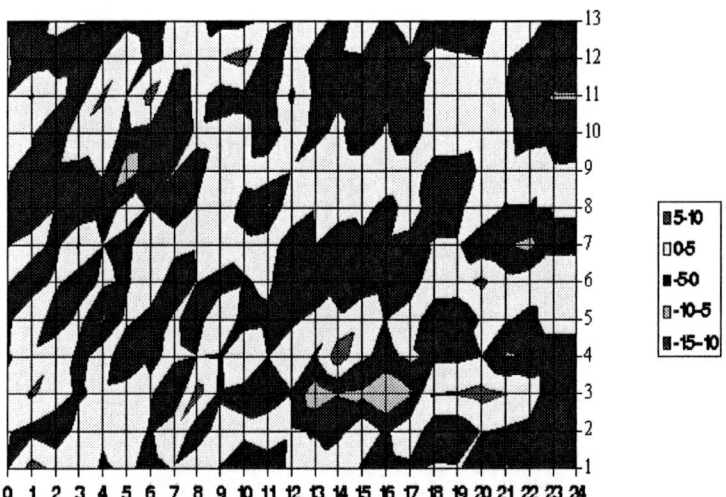

x-axis denote input and y-axis hidden Neurons

Figure 4.14: Synapses' Weights (600th Cycle)

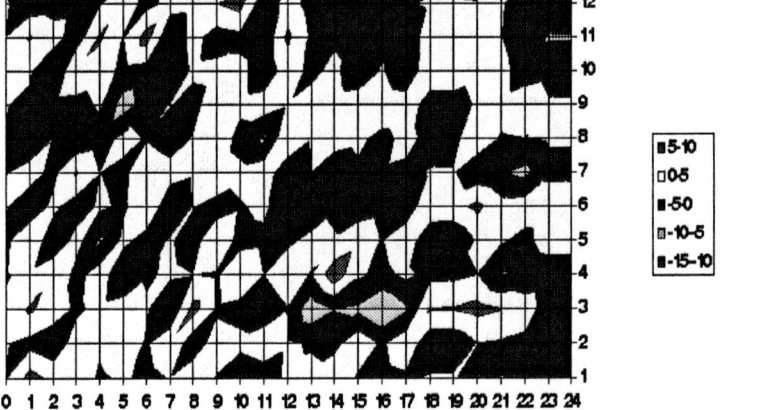

Figure 4.15: Synapses' Weights (750th Cycle)

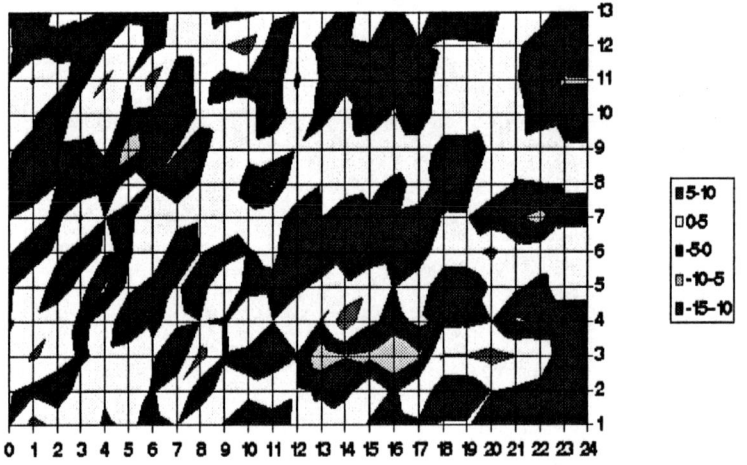

Figure 4.16: Synapses' Weights (900th Cycle)

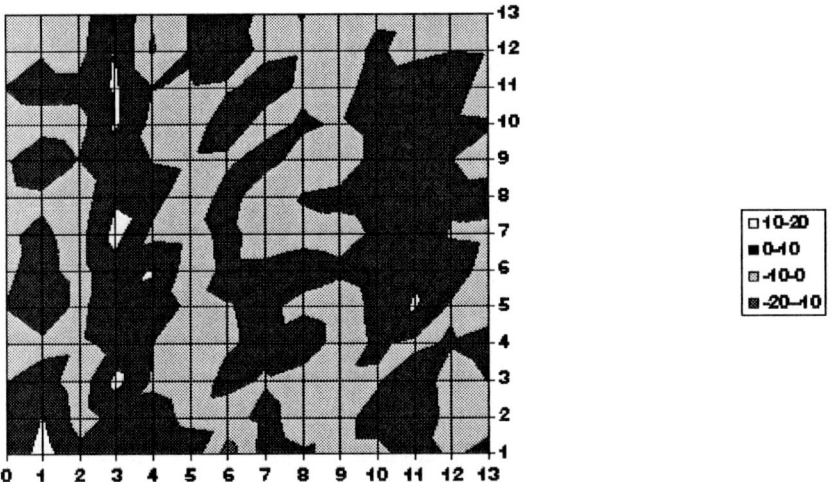

x-axis denote hidden and y-axis output Neurons

Figure 4.17: Synapses' Weights (150th Cycle)

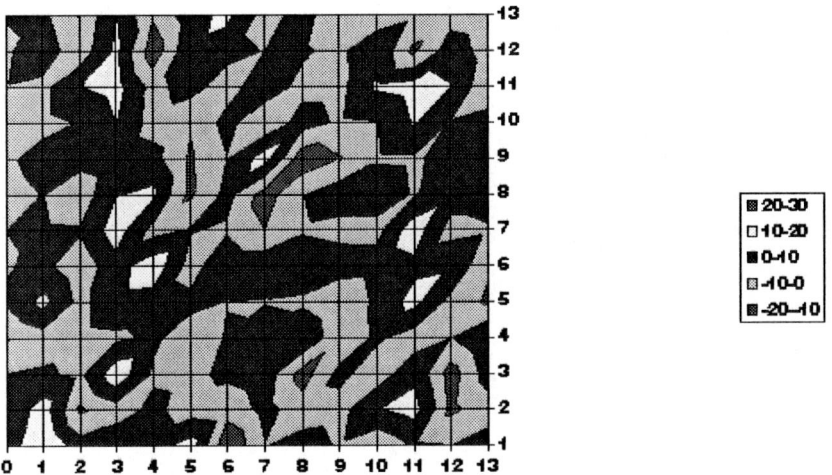

x-axis denote hidden and y-axis output Neurons

Figure 4.18: Synapses' Weights (300th Cycle)

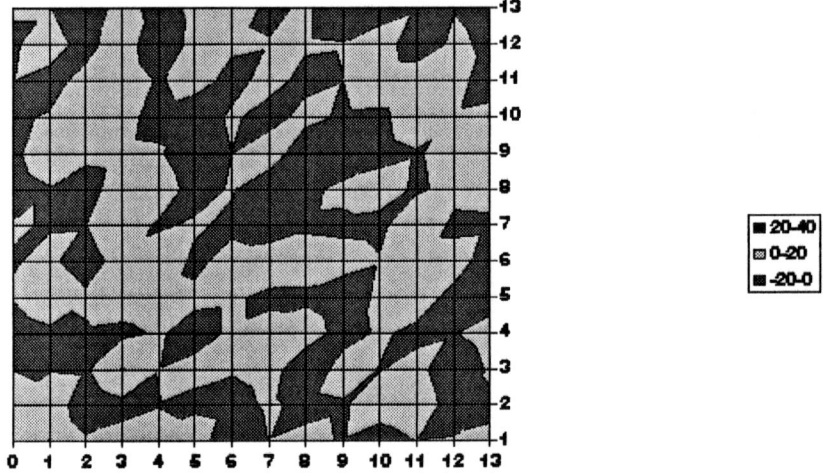

x-axis denote hidden and y-axis output Neurons

Figure 4.19: Synapses' Weights (450th Cycle)

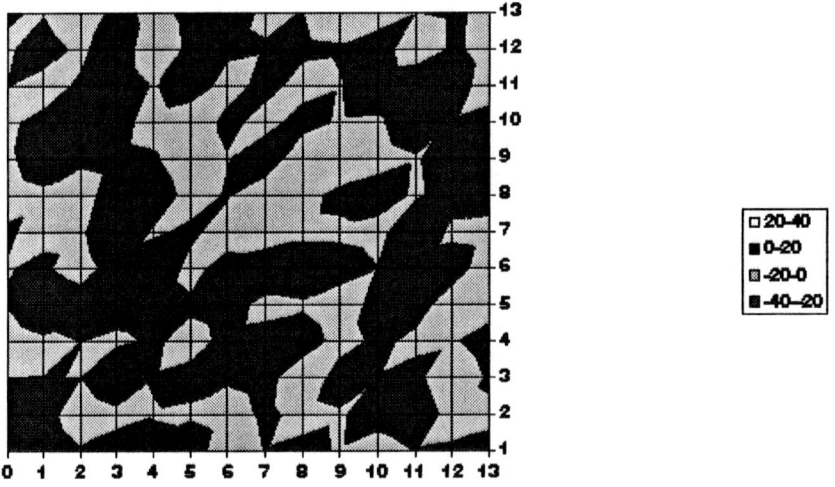

x-axis denote hidden and y-axis output Neurons

Figure 4.20: Synapses' Weights (600th Cycle)

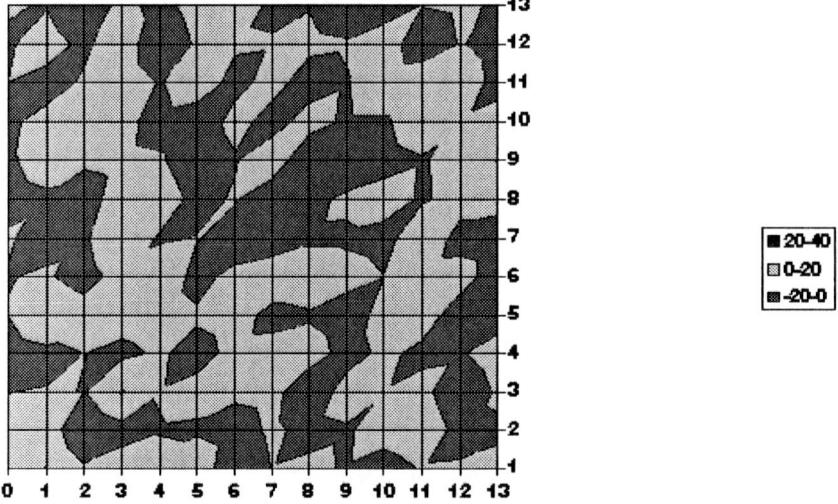

x-axis denote hidden and y-axis output Neurons

Figure 4.21: Synapses' Weights (750th Cycle)

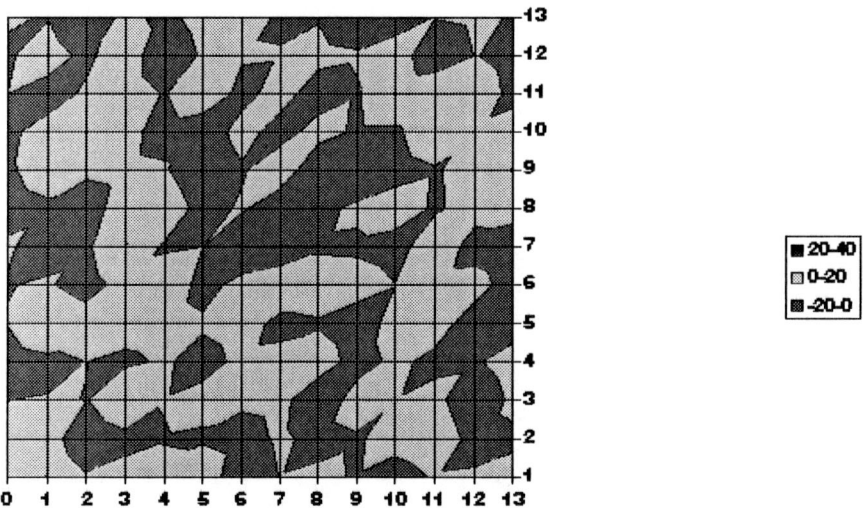

x-axis denote hidden and y-axis output Neurons

Figure 4.22: Synapses' Weights (900th Cycle)

a) **Zeroing** all the Weights whose physical value is "0" or near it, in order to decrease their number. The actual meaning for this action is that those Weights "carry" inputs to other Neurons (link them) that contribute little or nothing to a Neurons' response operation (firing). However, should this Neuron be implemented in software, no changes to its Network's size would be effective; it is by its implementation in hardware that smaller **external memory** would be needed [§6.5], or its Network's fit in an integrated chip of **smaller dimensions**, as well as into **reduced routing** of micro electronic circuitry in this chip.

b) To validate a successful **Weight initialization** procedure, especially backed up by the positive results of re-using their previous values reached when training the same ANN with some more or less Neurons. During the upgrade of an FFA-ANN to another, with a larger number of inputs or outputs, the experiments have shown that is not always necessary to re-initialize the Network and start the learning from the beginning. The same holds true for a downgrade of an FFA-ANN to another with a larger number of I/O.

c) **"Flattening"** more some valleys and **"raising"** more some hills between Learning Cycles, to achieve a faster convergence. Even preliminary experiments in benchmarking learning problems considering ANNs' use (e.g. hand-written symbols recognition), showed that the final neural convergence's course could be anticipated by observing an ANN's few initial Cycles Weights' evolution.

d) **Expanding** the previous rule in a neighboring area of grouped points showing a valley or hill. This is supported by the fact that the former suggest uniform, generally small contribution, and the latter represent powerful local decision paths; also those configurations **do not depend on each other** [Lip87].

e) Finally, some ANN's learning dominant rule "the winner takes it all" [§1.6], can be applied even in Weights' changes, i.e. some Synapses can be chosen to be preserved over other ones that are set aside. This can be done as long as these Weights adapt depending on the total effects of their neighborhood on the response of their local Neuron (e.g. their values fluctuate smoothly during the Learning Period) and the generalization of that rule to other Weights follows a successive course of topologic evolution in the whole ANN's architecture.

4.9 Conclusion

A methodology for solving the problem of using partial Learning Patterns is proposed, along with their re-forming to better suit particular input elements' responding behavior. It is referring to one of the most common problems the researchers face during the ANNs' learning: How the partial Patterns can be combined to form I/O vectors. The "Form-2" of Patterns mapping, proposes the application of a new methodology of input and output Patterns mapping, that evolves from output-centred to input-centred.

The use of a triadic logic in the elements mapping of input Patterns during the FFA-ANNs' learning is also proposed. The "Form-2" shapes the Learning Patterns by their input data (after the processing to their representation [§2.3]). Special factors can be given to the input vectors' elements; thus they can be further highlighted. The insertion of pseudo-inputs in the Learning Patterns leads to the total balance of the classes that are differentiated by FFA-ANNs and creates the reserving conditions for the future supply of new actual elements (e.g. new findings) without having to re-train the whole ANN or decision support system.

The number of hidden Slabs and Neurons and the special importance of Synapses' Weights were also studied. A hidden Slab is usually sufficient while hidden Neurons' number is defined by starting from a few and increasing them during the Learning Period. Conclusions drawn when intervening in Synapses' Weights during or after the ANN's convergence concern specific experimented cases and are applied by heuristic rules. The successful use of ANNs depends on the quality of the Learning Patterns and the correlations of data that they imply.

Finally, the application of heuristic or other rules in order to obtain an "optimized" procedure for defining hidden Neurons' number and Slabs constitutes an active research area. The herein presented schemes and the aforementioned results should be tested further and in more general applications.

4.10 References

[Lip87]   Lippmann, R. P., "An Introduction to Computing with NN", IEEE ASSP Magazine, vol. 5, pp. 4-22, 1987.

[M&C89] Mirchandani, G. and Cao, W., On Hidden Nodes for Neural Nets, IEEE Tans. on C&S, vol. 36, pp. 661-664, 1989.

[T&P89]   Touretzky, D. S. and Pomerlau, D. A., What's Hidden in the Hidden Layers?, Byte, vol. 14(8), pp. 227-233, 1989.

[HYH90] Hirose, Y., Yamashita, K., and Hijiya, S., Back-Propagation Algorithm which Varies the Number of Hidden Units, Neural Networks, vol. 4, pp. 61-66, 1990.

[L&L91]   Lin, C.-T. and Lee, C. S. G., Neural-Network-Based Fuzzy Logic Control and Decision System, IEEE Trans. on Comp., vol. 40, pp. 1320-1336, 1991.

[Pol91]   Poli, R., Cagnoni, S., Livi, R., Coppini, G., and Valli, G., "An NN Expert System for Diagnosing and Treating Hypertension", IEEE Comp., vol. 24, pp. 64-71, 1991.

[S&C91]   Schneider, C., and Card, H., "Analog CMOS Synaptic Learning Circuits Adapted from Invertebrate Biology", IEEE Trans. on C&S, vol. 38, pp. 1430-1438, 1991.

[C&T94] Cairns, G., and Tarassenko, L., "Learning with Analogue VLSI MLPs", Proc. of the 4th International Conference on Microelectronics for Neural Networks and Fuzzy Systems, Torino, Italy, pp. 67-76, Sep. 1994.

[H&P94] Hollis, P. and W., Paulos, J. J., "A Neural Network Learning Algorithm Tailored for VLSI Implementation", IEEE Trans. on NN, vol. 5, pp. 784-791, 1994.

[MMC94] Moreno, J. M., Madrenas, J., and Cabestany, J., "Systolic Modular VLSI Architecture for Multi-Model Neural Network Implementation", Proc. of the 4th International Conference on Microelectronics for Neural Networks and Fuzzy Systems, Torino, Italy, pp. 118-124, Sep. 1994.

[E94]   Economou, G. - P. K., Economopoulos, N. M., Charokopos, N., Zikos, P., Lymberopoulos, D., Spiropoulos, K., and Goutis, C. E., "Suggesting Diagnosis of Diseases and Treatment: How far Artificial Neural Networks can go?", Proc. of 1994 IEEE ISANN, Tainan, Taiwan, Dec. 1994.

[E95 I]   Economou, G. - P. K., Economopoulos, N. M., Lymberopoulos, D., and C. E. Goutis, "Experiences Accumulated Working towards Medical Decision Support Systems", J. of Microprocessing and Microprogramming, vol. 40, pp. 883-886, 1995.

[E95 II] Economou, G. - P. K., Lymberopoulos, D., and Goutis, C. E., "An ANNs-based System for the Diagnosis and Treatment of Diseases", Neural Processing Letters, vol. 2(1), pp. 22 -26, 1995.

5th Chapter

Implementation of the MDSS in Hardware

Once you write quality software,
you can adapt its algorithms to anything
Blaze Sima

5.1 Introduction

The work on the (Medical) Decision Support Systems would not be complete without a study dealing with their implementation in hardware. As it has already been mentioned [§3.11], the portability of these Systems in their most exploiting form remains the main challenge of this book, so a hardware design that would permit operation speed, extensibility, and adaptability was also sought.

This search was directed towards the development of the Medical System in hardware architectures and the sorting of parameters that would permit the arrangement of model Systems for a large number of applications. On the other hand, the appropriate factors for the preservation of the results obtained in the area of medicine should be ensured. New ANNs' aggregating topologies were re-examined and their effectiveness are herein extensively analyzed.

Hence, the idea of building a complete Medical System is promoted. It will be based on the already proposed structure and it could be easily altered to fit whatever cognitive field depending on any future medical need.

5.2 The Implementation in Hardware

Throughout the past chapters of this book, the DSS development underwent a thorough analysis concerning its implementation in software. The structures of its Neurons, their Networks and the System's and the methodologies that are related to its learning procedures were developed using the C programming language [§2.7, §4.2|7|8]. Some advantages were highlighted, such as **development easiness**, **direct supervision** of its processing, and when operating, **fairly quick responses**.

Our results up to now mainly constitute a first occurrence in areas that are well defined by an expert. The standardization of the input data, the identification of all correlations, and their proper feeding to the System was needed; though, more complicated fields, whereupon human experience is again dominant for the making of crucial decisions, call for larger **processing rates**. Moreover, **learning** and **continuous adaptation** in new applications' structures, required even in real time, ought to be confronted by fast Systems. This is what hardware ensures.

Likewise, other reasons also promote the System's implementation in hardware. The software **protection** from illegal copies, a main problem of software houses, is faced by using "locks" of hardware that accompanies a product and are "plugged in" the computers. These often delay the host computer's performance, conflict with its existing hardware, or demand the development of special software for their control. The System's full implementation in hardware smoothes all these glitches, and demands less specialized software components.

The non-existence of basic knowledge and proper utilization of computational systems in hospitals worldwide, usually discourage the utilization of specialized software products. The implementation in hardware offers an easy integration of the System in a package, satisfies the **size** and **transferability** demands, and results in its effective **standardization**. The above raise the System's implementation cost, but here follows a proposed methodology for the System's integration on silicon that ensures the **re-use** of its structures.

5.3 General Observations Concerning the Novel System

After the second Medical System was implemented [§3.9], the need for controlling the MDSS' effectiveness was replaced by developing it onto a more general application basis. This was characterized by operations' speed and adaptation in different areas of human expertise - the reasons behind its hardware re-design. Thus, a series of specifications for its implementation had to be set.

The design of a **general architecture** for the implementation in hardware is also demanded for practical reasons. This architecture should permit the data definition and their (ANN) aggregation depending on the application. The segregation of a more general system in FFA-ANN interconnected groups, according to a proper architecture, applies to other fields, too. The problem is to ensure data transfer along these Networks, a topic that reflects in the developing of many conduits among silicon processing elements (gates) and of a **large chip area**. This difficulty is faced with the non-simultaneous implementation of all the System's Neurons (therefore of Networks too) [§2.6].

The System's **adaptation** in the application structures is achieved through the proper ANNs' architecture. The projection of human experience on their Synapses primarily constitutes a mapping problem of input data - faced already with procedures mentioned [§4.4]. During the implementation in hardware, ensuring the handling of the Weights (that arise from the ANNs teaching) was another goal set. These specifications are met by first teaching the ANNs in software [§5.11].

The System integration in silicon also poses the problem of choosing its **design method**. The digital and analog circuits present intrinsic advantages and disadvantages but the same stands also for the available **design, control,** and **fabrication** tools that are available [Dis91, Eur93]. A digital data circuit was chosen, as the existing technology covers the demands and because it permits the utilization of general design structures, as it will be shown next.

5.4 Approximation of the Artificial Neuron

A large part of an ANN's ability to converge to its Learning Patterns is due to the Sigmoid function that undertakes the processing of the weighted factors that a Neuron accepts (Fig. 1.1, 5.1). Its non-linearity leads ANNs to **emulate** the biological neurons [Lip87], accomplish **mathematical constraints** [T&H86], and their **state trajectory** towards lower energy levels (convergence) [Hop88].

Researchers proposed many forms of the Sigmoid, mainly as shown [§1.2]:

$$\varphi(\zeta) = \text{sign}(\zeta), \; \varphi(\zeta) = \frac{1}{1+e^{-\zeta-\Pi}}, \; \varphi(\zeta) = \frac{1-e^{-\alpha*\zeta}}{1+e^{-\alpha*\zeta}},$$

(5.1 a, b, c)

Each one is followed by a learning algorithm. With the only exception of the back propagation rule, more applied along to Eq. 5.1b (see Fig. 5.1(a); it uses other forms of Sigmoids), no-one **general** form has prevailed, mainly because of this function's adaptation to the demands of each learning algorithm.

Usually, its **smooth continuity** in the field where the Learning Patterns are derived is required (existence of its **first derivative** and, less often also, of its **second derivative**). Its characteristic equation affects the **convergence**, the **speed**, and the **accuracy** of learning algorithms, as proven by the experiments in software and mathematical analysis [Lip87].

Moreover, its form is also defined by **numerical accuracy norms**. As it is a function that can be approximated by non-terminating decimal numerals, the choice of its appropriate numerical mapping crucially affects all the calculations.

In order to implement the proposed MDSS in hardware, the approximation of the Sigmoid with a piece-wise linear function of the same upper and lower limits (logical "0"s and "1"a) and a local gradient slope having the value of 2^{-4} was used [E94 I]. Fig. 5.1a represents the software experiments Sigmoid [S&T92] (also represented in Eq. 5.1c), and its piece-wise linearly approximated form (Fig. 5.1b).

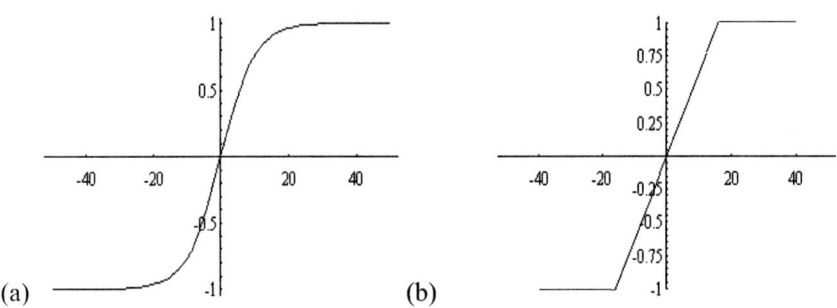

Figure 5.1: The Two Sigmoid Functions

Software experiments being conducted on the same medical applications have shown that also with this approximation of their Sigmoid, the ANNs **converged** to the same Learning Patterns. Consequently, the medical data that determine the diagnosis flow have indeed been classified into separate classes so as the symptoms and their findings lead univocally to the diseases (and treatment).

Moreover, the **diagnosis accuracy** of the Medical System had not changed. This was true because it was demanded by the Networks to converge to the same convergence error (1% or less). In case where the norms were not satisfied, the experiment would be judged as failed and the approximation would change.

The ANNs **convergence time** with the new Sigmoid was larger, i.e. 5 - 10% more. This ascertainment could be characterized as predictable should the Network's complexity be taken into account. Overall, the Sigmoid constitutes the main factor for the differentiation of the created classification sub-fields [§4.6] and its approximation affects their creation process.

Furthermore, the difference between a Network's outputs increased, therefore the **distinctness's diversification** between the diseases [§3.8.2] enlarged as the use of the piece-wise linear Sigmoid augmented the discrimination up to 8 - 12%. The curve form of the Sigmoid ensures better smoothness of its values.

The ANN was more easily **implemented** in software. The multiplication to a constant (linear parts of the new Sigmoid) is much more easy for a computer than the use of the exponential function (necessary element of the Sigmoid, Eq. 5.1).

The rather predictable results should be attributed to the field's classification performed by the ANNs' mapping. Since the presence of more hidden layers than 1 for the proper operation of the Medical System was not demanded (§3.8.2], the alteration to the Sigmoid could not bring about big changes.

The used numerical accuracy of the implementation was also a research topic. During the software programming of ANNs' performance, it was initially kept on the maximum possible by using **double floating-point arithmetic**. It was observed, however, that the Weights' numerical value in their Synapses in different ANNs **spanned** between minima of -50.0 up to maxima of +50.0 [E94 I].

More adaptation changes in the **form** of the piece-wise linear Sigmoid were also studied. Specialized local region approximations and linear sections with other gradient values were tested in different points with the purpose of finding how many different values and to which intervals would best fit the actual Sigmoid. Moreover, the proposed interventions in the Network learning procedure [§4.6|7|8] were analyzed by means of these approximations approximations.

Our conclusions are that more piece-wise linear sections with other gradients or even local approximations do not essentially add to the approximated Sigmoid's performance. Furthermore, the **alteration** of the used **numerical accuracy** would not affect the total performance of the Medical Systems or of the other applications. The gradient was fit to the value of 2^{-4} and the value of Weights (after the ANNs' convergence, as it was already been achieved in software) was reduced to the **8-bit fixed-point arithmetic**.

The proper projection of a problem's variables in the ANNs' Learning Patterns solves a large part of all problems and ensures a satisfying operation. In sort, ANNs are taught in software with the actual Sigmoid's form, whereas allowed full numerical double floating-point accuracy for their Weights. They are used, though, with the piece-wise linear approximated Sigmoid form and the reduced Weights' values, traits - also transferred in their hardware design.

5.5 Use of the Field Programmable Gate Arrays

Beyond the speed advantages, the System's implementation in hardware, as an autonomous unit, permits its use away from organized and fully equipped medical centers. Sometimes an MD has to visit a patient in his/her residence and/or in a remote area with scarce or limited resources.

One of the disadvantages of using application-specific integrated circuits (ASICs) is due to the high development cost and small re-adjustment capability of their data interfaces. The utilization of the field programmable gate arrays (FPGAs) guarantees that new ANNs' topologies will be defined on the System under evolution without costly changes in their hardware part [Xil98].

Moreover, the already-developed Medical Systems can be considered as one, since they have experimentally been given the same ANNs' **topology**, the use of the **CDDM** to their operation flows, and the same **environment** of **local connections** for their Networks. The two MDSSs integrate into one with the simulation of a general System's architecture that alternates its application area in pulmonary, haematology etc. diseases, by the use of the proper Weights.

The one problem that could restrict the whole effort is determined by their nature: FPGAs constitute **digital implementations of discrete time data**. ANNs that have been so far exploited, though, constitute processing elements of **analog data of continuous time**. However, they have been emulated in a computer.

The lack of ANNs' feedback connections (Neuron Synapses towards their feeding Neurons) in FFA-ANNs also permits the independent **consideration of each Neuron** [Fig. 1.1]. The multiplication of Weights and inputs, the summation of the partial products, and the results being processed by the Sigmoid, correspond to operations that accept no other influence than their inputs. Hence, they can be partitioned in time into distributed operations, if demanded during the implementation or the System's design, by using a different approach.

The FFA-ANN also permits the **storage** of the intermediate Neurons' results of a given Network so that they can be used later on. These memory units could also be placed out of an FPGA (and definitely inside an integrated circuit, in the future). The realization of **different ANNs** in different time slots, also occurs by the use of FFA-ANNs. In real time, the FPGAs will be programmed to be specific ANNs and their inputs and outputs connections will come along too.

Therefore, the **partition in time** of the operating, approximated Neurons, ANNs, and the of the whole Medical System for its implementation by means of FPGAs, is proposed. External memories will provide the Neurons to be implemented Synapses' Weights, and will store their intermediate results.

5.6 Implementation's Structure

Following the previous analysis, the units that will implement the System in the proposed FPGA architecture are described. These will complete the Neurons, the storage of Weights and intermediate results, and the communication protocol.

The last does not constitute a design problem. The asynchronous communication by means of a serial gate establishes a trusted model of data transmission with a satisfying performance. Chips of extended market use integrate it and the serial gate constitutes a model input in many computational systems.

Fig. 5.2 represents the proposed architecture.

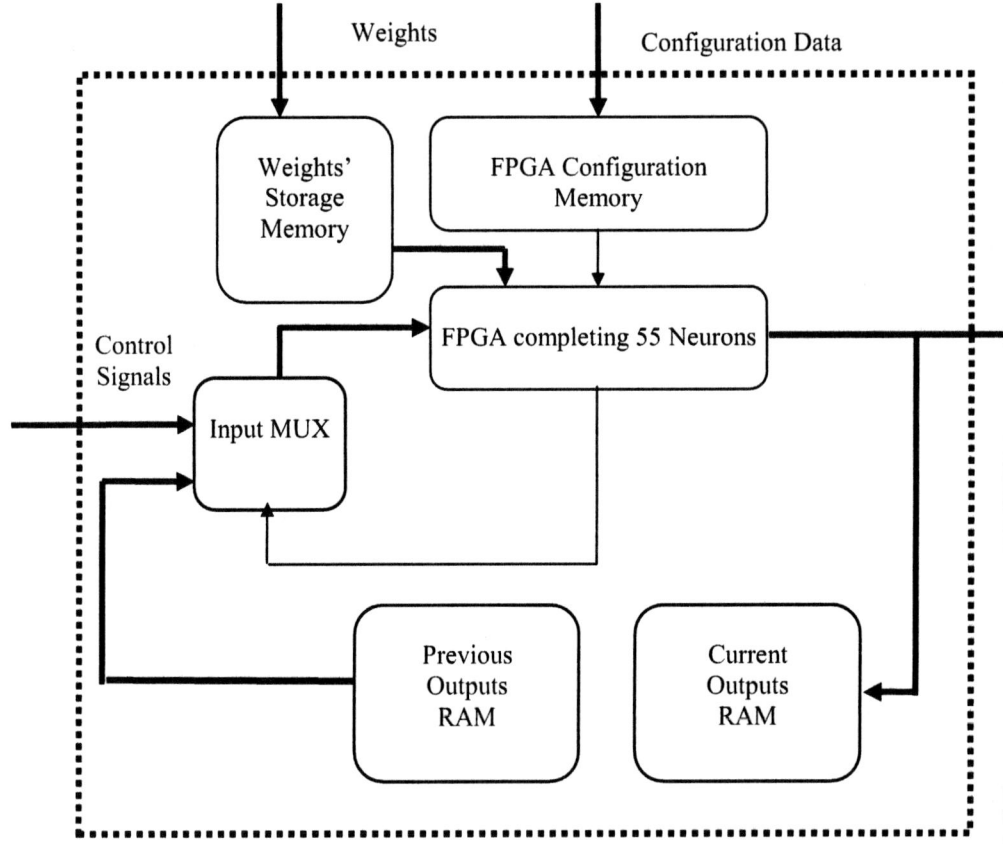

Figure 5.2: System's Units Connections

5.7 The Implemented Neuron
The operations of multiplication, summation and convolution (through the Sigmoid) constitute the functioning basis of every Neuron [§1.2]. Its operation generally obeys the following equation [Sib93]:

$$\psi = \varphi(\sum_{i=1}^{n} \beta_{ij} * \psi'_i - \Pi_j) \tag{5.2}$$

ψ, ψ' denote the Neuron's input and output, while Π, a possible biased input

Thus, the System's hardware design presupposes the discretization of the above operations as well as their execution by digital components; summation can be executed by serial **accumulators** or with **parallel Wallace trees** [Hwa79].

For the calculation in parallel of the Weights multiplications to the corresponded Neuron inputs, a large number of identical units would be needed.

Yet, a **multiplier - accumulator topology** was chosen that accepts inputs serially, multiplies, and sums them up into a **register** - also achieving the result's storage.

The Sigmoid is approximated as aforementioned, having a linear section with a gradient of value 2^{-4} and saturators when logical "0" or "1" is needed.

Fig. 5.3 shows the implemented Neuron.

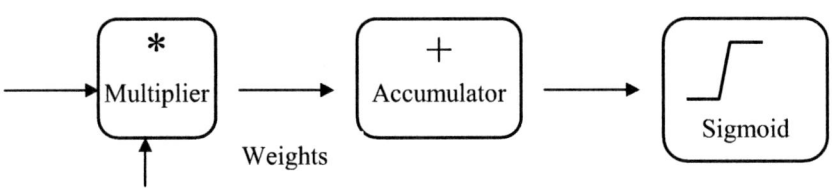

Figure 5.3: Implemented Neuron

5.8 Neuron's Design

The three modules depicted in Fig. 5.3 are herein covered in more details. Their proposed architecture satisfies the **space norm** set by the FPGA as their manufacturer (XILINX) imposes [Xil98]. More specifically, eight is the maximum number of Neurons implemented; they can cover the System's demands with their continuous re-utilization [§5.5].

Although almost the whole surface of FPGAs is exploited, it can **fast** process the inputs' data. All the other necessary design features, such as the **ANNs' mapping**, correctly corresponding the ANNs' **Weights**, and the **storage** of their intermediate results (by using of external memories) have been devised to be done quickly with the use of market components.

This architecture boosts very good, **repetitive** use of all the existing circuit components. Special care has been taken for their **proper clocking**.

5.8.1 The Proposed Multiplier-Adder/Accumulator

Fig. 5.4 shows the proposed unit. It handles bit-serial data, so as to save size.

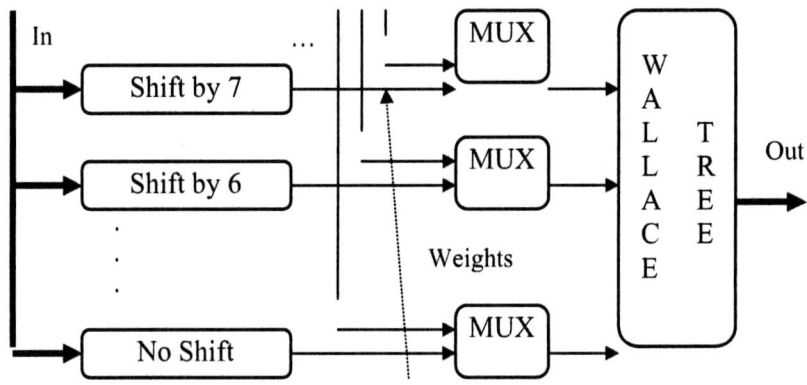

Figure 5.4: The Proposed Multiplier - Adder/Accumulator

It is a relatively simple topology that permits:
- The insertion of eight (8) bit fixed-point arithmetic digits, a bit per time. In that way, exploitation is made of a serial input in a parallel process.
- The simultaneous shifting of these digits. A multiplexer (Fig. 5.4, "MUX") unit, allow for their multiplication to the appropriate Weight.
- The pipeline processing as is below explained.

Fig. 5.5 depicts the time course of the digits of a 3-digit number ($\gamma_0\beta_0\alpha_0$) through the shift components. For simplicity, the multiplexer is not shown and the shifters have been degenerated into 1-digit delays.

The multiplexers that "multiply" the Weights to the incoming digits are not depicted in Fig. 5.5. They are placed before the adder and, as all incoming digits have been normalized in the [0, 1] interval, they mainly degrade the input values. Pipelining is used to avoid speed reduction that might be caused by bit-serial arithmetic. Since the MS digits of the shifted values are always constant "0" or "1" and equal to the MS digit of the original number, they cannot be used. Thus, shifting of the next input value starts before multiplication of the previous one has finished. This multiplier was estimated to occupy about eighteen (18) Configurable Logic Blocks (CLBs) of the XILINX XC4062XL FPGA [Xil98].

The implementation's delay is the result of the shifted digits carriage to the adder. Despite this, since digits are represented as two's complement, the first digit that exits after the shifting of the MS one is the MS digit itself. Therefore, it is known *a priori*, so it can be foretold and be placed to the adder, 2 operating cycles in advance [Fig. 5.5], seven (7) cycles in advance for the 8-bits application.

The accumulator unit is composed by a serial digits adder that handles numbers of 8 digits, plus a corresponding register.

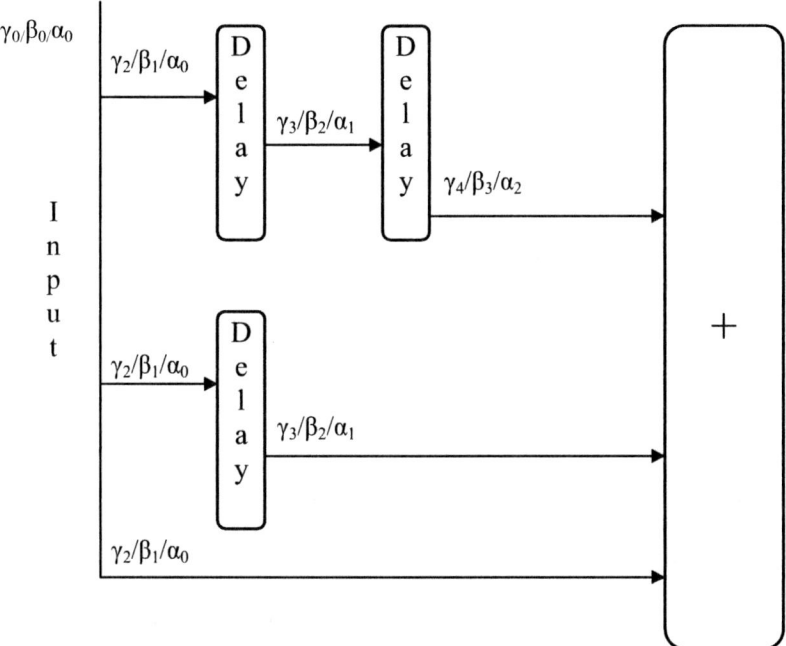

Figure 5.5: A 3-digit Number throughout the Multiplier - Adder/Accumulator

5.8.2 Numerical Representation and Sigmoid

The circuit that undertakes the Sigmoid function's approximation is composed by simple circuits and mainly by a comparator/saturator (for cutting off the input to the laid limits), a shifter of 4 digits (that implements the 2^{-4} gradient), and a multiplexer. The comparator feeds the control input of the multiplexer allowing for its output to be "0", "1" or the shifted input's value, (constituted by the summation of the Weights' products to the actual inputs). Fig. 5.6 shows this circuit.

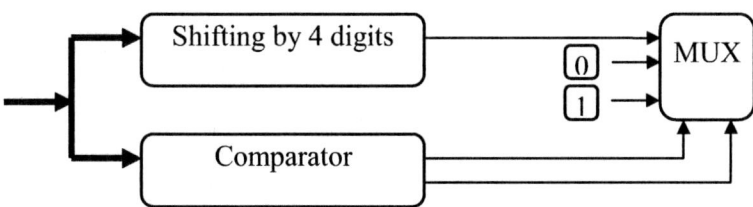

Figure 5.6: The Sigmoid Function's Approximation

5.9 Implementation's Important Features

Input data's accuracy was set to 8 bits, a value obtained experimentally. A 7 bits accuracy might also be adequate for the specific application; the use of 8 bits has been decided in order to be compatible with possible future applications.

On the other hand, the design of the Medical System in FPGA, taking under consideration the speed specifications and the chip size, reached a compromise: the serial (and not parallel) operation of some of the ANNs' Synapses. This can be without problems exercised as the FFA-ANN depends on the response of each of its Neuron by separately calculating the contribution of their previous nodes.

As a consequence, each FPGA will include 55 identical Neurons, at most. A parallel input-serial output register transfers the inputs from the external memory to the Synapses, while a multiplexer unit will sort through the addresses of Neurons output values storing them in the same memory (from where they will be recalled by following the same procedure, by the next Slab [§1.2]).

A control module that monitors the execution of the entire structure (not shown), can also be integrated in the FPGA. Yet, to allow for possible increase in the complexity (and thus in the size) of the control module, the use of a second FPGA chip could be considered. Still, this approach bears no further complexity.

The whole MDSS will be composed by the FPGA(s), the RAM for intermediate store of ANNs' outputs, and the Weights storage memory. The proposed system structure is shown in Fig. 5.7. Two more elements are present: the input MUX, that is used to select inputs for the FPGA module either from previous results or from the user; and the RAM that holds the configuration bit stream.

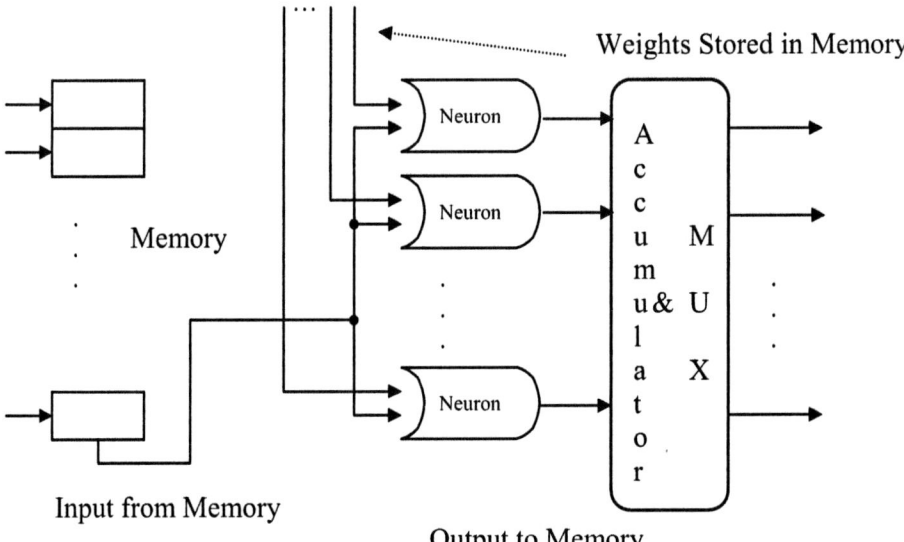

Figure 5.7: FPGA's Contents

5.10 Definition of an Application's Parameters

Developing facilities for the system's update is crucial. First, in the case any new data needs to be fed, and second, should a new system's structure be developed. A powerful computer can be used at a medical center that would eventually train the MDSS with new medical data. The outcome Weights can be stored in a file.

Similarly, the development of a new structure that will either enhance the existing MDSS or add new capabilities to it (consider more symptoms, etc.), should pass through a phase where Learning Patterns would be developed, the System's structure would be simulated, etc. When the results show that it can be used in practical situations, a designer will have to make an FPGA prototype (using the tools of XILINX) and prepare a configuration bit stream file.

Both files can be then loaded on the System via magnetic storage media or even through the Internet or by by using eMAIL communication protocols.

Fig. 5.8 shows a schematic representation for this procedure.

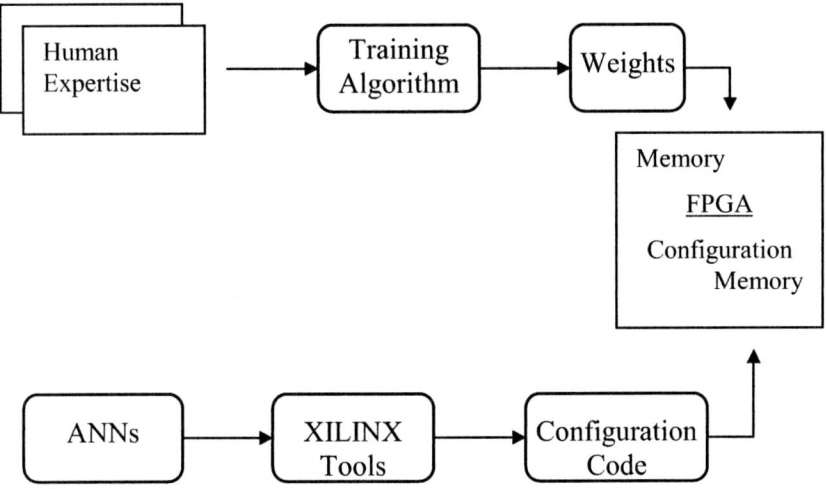

Figure 5.8: MDSS Updating Procedure Scheme

5.11 A Comparison of the Novel Implementation's Traits

In the bibliography, the trend dominating the ANNs use in all the applications that have already been described [§1.9] is the satisfaction of their specifications having no special demands for their generalization in software or hardware. This also constitutes the main request in the development of methodologies for solving problems by means of ANNs, so the development and evolution of complicated Networks or learning algorithms must not become an end in itself, when even more simple ANNs perform very well according to the set norms. Under this approximation, most of the implementations in hardware are not characterized by the development generality but by the construction specialization.

Some of these implementation categories are:
- ANNs of **Digital/Analog** circuits. The implementation of the first concerns smart techniques for handling memory demands [Dis 91]; the second's demands do not differentiate from the general analog design problem [Vit94].
- ANNs with an **embedded learning algorithm**. They are chips that include special construction techniques [LSY91], or they exploit approximations of artificial neural networks learning algorithms [H&P94].
- ANNs being integrated **older Networks** that had been implemented in software [W&E92]. In a way they supply a more appropriate implementation environment, mainly by the point of the speed considerations.
- ANNs that are destined to be used as **(pre-)processors** in more general systems. The design emphasis is given on the chips' communication [NN92].
- ANNs that are developed in specialized architectures - emphasis to be given on their **operational behavior** (mapping of data) [HVK89].

A number of more special ANNs' chips are focused on the calculation of parameters for the construction of other ANNs [Per91]. Such applications are usually based on the Hopfield's analog ANN [Hop88], [§1.5].

Moreover, ANN implementations differ in **analog applications** (signal converters from analog to digital [T&H86]), memories [Far85], image recognition [N&C92] and in realizing the system of automatic control of **artificial arms** [S&F94]. These implementations, however, offer solutions that are mainly applied on a series of **similarly-defined problems** or **applications**.

Furthermore, they do not work on the problem of **redefining** a Network's application field. The newer application updates are usually redesigned from zero-base and are reintegrated in silicon. All the same, they design the chip so as to focus towards a single **ANN architecture**. Other ANNs implementations in hardware can be found in a surplus of publications and conference papers [NN92, 93, Eur93].

The new architecture design of the Decision Support System with the proposed implementation in silicon shows many advantages, such as the adaptation **flexibility** in a great number of applications. The implemented Neurons rely on the operator, who will decide about their connections (Synapses). In that way not only can the specific FFA-ANN or the System be implemented, but also a significant number of other Networks. By defining the FPGA configuration and by providing for the appropriate Weights, the Neuron topology, the ANNs architecture, and whatever System's structure are promptly implemented.

The **type and approximation** of the Sigmoid can vary as is mapped on a series of specialized shifters - offering another implementation advantage. In that way, more "gradient areas", even different kinds of Sigmoids, can be implemented in the same ANN. The Sigmoid's approximation accuracy depends only on the application and is not limited by the FPGA configuration.

The downloading of the Weights' values (as they are reached from the Networks' learning in other computational systems), permits the decrease of learning time and the achievement of the needed accuracy. During this procedure the presence of a specialized developer is not demanded. Thus, the demand for incorporating the learning algorithm in the chip is properly faced.

On the other hand, the proposed implementation does not offer an extremely new design. The originality of the architecture, though, consists in the re-use of its structures and the easy definition of the operation of the approximated Networks.

The MDSS has also been described in the VHDL hardware design language for both prototyping back-up and ensuring future portability to any VLSI design rules technology reasons. This topic is fully detailed in the next sections.

5.12 Parametrical Hardware Design

The implementation in FPGA of the new Decision Support System has already been analyzed. Beyond its smaller (maybe) operating speed in relation to other designs, it is accompanied by a series of restrictions that concern its basis of implementation. The design of a circuit should fulfill the particular design rules that a manufacturer imposes and is "tied" to the utilized design tool. Also, its efficiency is determined to a great extent by the implementation technology.

This issue will be confronted by the use of a model hardware description language; thus the design will be free of any restrictions posed by the use of a particular design tool. In other words, the System was also implemented by means of the hardware description language for Very Large Scale Integrated Circuits (VHDL). The capabilities of this hardware description language guarantee the independence from the manufacturer and from the design tools, rendering the architecture of the specific Medical System variably implemented [Coe89].

The hardware description language VHDL is also based on standardized structures. It can take into account a chip's characteristics by its layout [Lee92].

5.13 ANNs' Design Using the VHDL Language

VHDL [Std88] provides independence from manufacturers and design tools alike, but on the other hand, when special circuits are not developed for it, it has disadvantages in operation speed [Ber92].

The VHDL language permits the thorough description of even special-purpose designs, step by step, or the building of a behavioral model to be used as a "black box" instead. In the second case, a standardized tool takes charge of the circuits' translation in the library of some manufacturers; therefore a decrease in speed.

For completeness reasons, a behavioral model of the MDSS components was developed. More specifically, the exploitation of the modules of many leaf cells (basic circuits in silicon) that are developed by different designers and are applied independently of the manufacturer was our main goal [E93 I]. By using VHDL, the designs transit in different manufacturers' technologies is done more easily [Nav93].

Furthermore, the VHDL language permits the design to enter into an environment where the description of a circuit response suffices from the emulation and its final implementation. In this way, it accommodates the retargeting of FFA-ANN's System and also the Networks themselves in different application structures. With the feeding of the appropriate parameters that are related to the connections of the Networks or their Neurons, to the corresponding sections of the implementation's code, a "new" System or ANNs capable to converge to other Learning Patterns are built. The language itself provides the appropriate experiments base.

Fig. 5.9 and 5.10 represents the code in a VHDL of a Neuron and Fig. 5.11 depicts the approximated Neuron (a modification of Fig. 5.3) [E95].

```
library IEEE;
use IEEE.std_logic_1164.all;

ENTITY Neuron IS
    PORT (R: in BIT; W: in INTEGER; I: in INTEGER; Wp: in BIT;
        MW: in BIT; MI: in BIT; O: out INTEGER);
END Neuron;
```

Figure 5.9: VHDL Behavioural Model of A Neuron (headers)

```
ARCHITECTURE behavioral OF Neuron IS
    SIGNAL INPUT: INTEGER;
    SIGNAL WEIGHT: INTEGER;
    SIGNAL PROSIG: INTEGER;
    SIGNAL AFTERSIG: INTEGER;

BEGIN
    O <= AFTERSIG;
    changes: PROCESS(MW, MI, PROSIG, W, I)
    BEGIN
        IF (MW = '0') THEN
            WEIGHT <= W;
        END IF;
        IF (MI = '0') THEN
            INPUT <= I;
        END IF;
        IF (PROSIG < -5) THEN
            AFTERSIG<=-10;
        END IF;
        IF (PROSIG > 5) THEN
            AFTERSIG <= 10;
        END IF;
        IF ( (PROSIG > -5) AND (PROSIG < 5) ) THEN
            AFTERSIG <= PROSIG*2;
        END IF;
    END PROCESS;
```

```
addition: PROCESS(R, Wp, MW, MI)
BEGIN
    IF ( (Wp= '1') AND (Wp'EVENT) ) THEN
        IF ( (MW = '1') AND (MI = '1')) THEN
            PROSIG <= PROSIG+WEIGHT*INPUT/100;
        END IF;
        IF (R = '0') THEN
            PROSIG < =0;
        END IF;
    END IF;
END PROCESS;
END behavioral;
```

Figure 5.10: VHDL Behavioural Model of A Neuron (body)

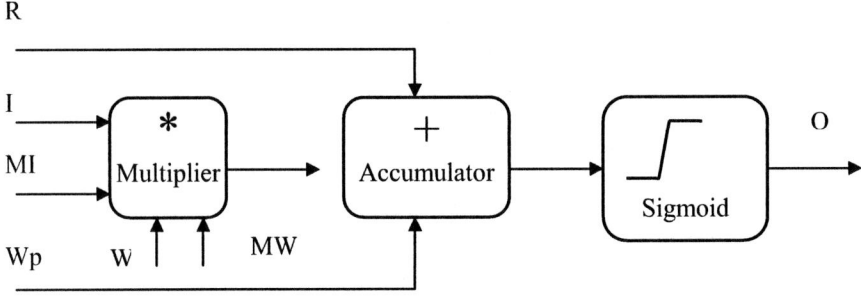

Figure 5.11: Implemented VHDL Neuron Model

The signals that are depicted in Fig 5.11 are:
- **I/O**, input/output word from/to previous/next Layer. This word is represented by means of 8-digit numbers [§5.9].
- **W**, input word for the feeding of Weights to the multiplier. They are also represented by means of eight 8-digit numbers [§5.9]
- **Wp**, input digit, the clock-pulse series for summations' synchronization.
- **MI/MW**, input digits that are used as the design's control inputs for the receipt of a novel input/Weight at time 0.
- **R**, input digit, causes the synchronous accumulator's reset.

The above VHDL code (Fig. 5.9, 5.10) satisfies the specifications for the easy representation of FFA-ANNs and during the emulation process (a tool given by a standardized VHDL design package) it can map to leaf cells data of any selected manufacturer. It is also characterized by the use of the structural programming so that even a less specialized designer can handle it. This code has also been optimized as parameters requiring less silicon area have been used (integers, bits).

5.14 Conclusion

The abilities of induction and generalization of the proposed DSS were decided to be enhanced by means of its implementation in hardware. The System design in an architecture of digital components and its implementation by means of FPGA CLBs were selected. The main reason supporting this implementation is the re-targeting of their structures (elements and connections) that FPGAs offer.

On the other hand, the demand for the design of the proposed System in hardware was met after a series of experiments that defined the **type** of the numerical data representation, the **approximation** of the Neurons' Sigmoid, and their appropriate implementation's **modules** by FPGAs. The experiments took place on the same computational environment where the medical applications were developed covering the implementation in software of FFA-ANNs with **piece-wise linear Sigmoid** of a researched gradient, **different** numerical representation **accuracy**, and the re-teaching of FFA-ANNs with combination of these changes.

The results showed that the System could be implemented with these changes and that the only differences in its performance were the **percentages** and not the **classification sequence of its outputs**. Also, the distinctive architecture of FFA-ANNs made the repetitive use of 55 approximated Neurons (the maximum number of Neurons the given FPGA holds) realize the whole Medical System.

With the implementation of the MDSS architecture in hardware, the necessary process speed is achieved. This feature constitutes the crucial factor for the transition of the System in more complicated applications fields, such as the combination of Medical Systems of different medical areas in one (e.g. pulmonology and otolaryngology, haematology and heart disorders etc.)

Another factor, the design's independence from a silicon manufacturer, was solved by the use of the VHDL language, since it ensures an integrated design environment for the DSS. In association with the easy retargeting of the FPGAs, it provides the System the ability to be implemented and tested in different platforms.

Furthermore, the approximation specifications of the artificial neuron, as they have been set herein, are incorporated into the code of the VHDL hardware description language and can be promptly adapted in whatever design demands that are related with a manufacturer's leaf cells, the implemented arithmetic operations, approximations of the Sigmoid, or different type of memories. The approximations fit in elements more orientated to ANNs utilization, i.e. different Neurons, architectures, can even be integrated as learning algorithms on a chip.

5.15 References

[Hwa79] Hwang, K., Computer Arithmetic: Principles, Architecture and Design, Wiley, New York, 1979.

[Far85] Farhat, N. H., Psaltis, D., Prata, A., and Paek, E., "Optical Implementation of the Hopfield Model", App. Opt., vol. 24, pp. 1469-1475, 1985.

[T&H86]	Tank, D. W. and Hopfield, J. J., "Simple "Neural" Optimization Networks: An A/D Converter, Signal Decision Circuit, and a Linear Programming Circuit", IEEE Trans. on C&S, vol. 33, pp. 533-541, 1986.
[Lip87]	Lippmann, R. P., "An Introduction to Computing with NN", IEEE ASSP Mag., vol. 5, pp. 4-22, 1987.
[Hop88]	Hopfield, J. J., "ANNs", Cir. & Dev. Mag., vol. 4(9), pp. 3-10, 1988.
[Std88]	IEEE Standard VHDL Language Reference Manual, IEEE, New York, 1988.
[Coe89]	Coelho, D. R., The VHDL Handbook, Kluwer, Boston, 1989.
[HVK89]	Hwang, J.-N., Vlontzos, J. A., and Kung, S.-Y., "A Systolic Neural Network Architecture for Hidden Markov Models", IEEE Trans. on ASSP, vol. 37, pp. 1967-1979, 1989.
[Dis91]	Distante, F., Sami, M., Stefanelli, R., and Storti-Gajani, G., "Mapping Neural Nets onto a Massively Parallel Architecture: A Defect-Tolerance Solution", Proc. of the IEEE, vol. 79, pp. 444-460, 1991.
[LSY91]	Lee, B. W., Sheu, B. J., and Yang, H., "Analog Floating-Gate Synapses for General-Purpose VLSI Neural Computation", IEEE Trans. on C&S, vol. 38, pp. 654-658, 1991.
[Per91]	Perfetti, R., "A Neural Network to Design Neural Networks", IEEE Trans. on C&S, vol. 38, pp. 1099-1103, 1991.
[Ber92]	Bergé, J.-M., Fonkoua, A., Magino, S., and Rouilland, J., VHDL '92: The new Features of the VHDL Hardware Description Language, Kluwer, Boston, 1992.
[Lee92]	Lee, C.-H., Digital System Design Using VHDL, CorralTek, Salinas, 1992.
[N&C92]	Nasrabadi, N. M. and Choo, C. Y., "Hopfield Network for Stereo Vision Correspondence", IEEE Trans. on NN, vol. 3, pp. 5-13, 1992.
[NN92]	"Special Issue on Neural Networks Hardware", IEEE Trans. on NN, vol. 3(3), 1992.
[S&T92]	Scalero, R. S. and Tepedelenlioglu, N., "A Fast New Algorithm for Training Feedforward NN", IEEE Trans. on Sig. Proc., vol. 40, pp. 202-210, 1992.
[W&E92]	White, B. A. and Elmasry, M. I.,"The Digi-Neocognitron": A Digital Neocognitron Neural Network Model for VLSI", IEEE Trans. on NN, vol. 3, pp. 73-85, 1992.
[Eur93]	Special Topics on ANN's Implementation, Proc. of the 19th EuroMicro Conference: Open System Design (Hardware, Software and Applications), Barcelona, Spain, 1993.
[Nav93]	Navabi, Z., VHDL: Analysis and Modeling of Digital Systems, McGraw-Hill, New York, 1993.
[NN93]	"Special Issue on Neural Networks Hardware", IEEE Trans. on NN, vol. 4(3), 1993.
[Sib93]	Sibai, F. N., "A Fault Tolerant Digital Artificial Neuron", IEEE Des. and Test of Comp., vol. 10(4), pp. 76-82, 1993.

[H&P94]   Hollis, P. W. and Paulos, J. J., "A Neural Network Learning Algorithm Tailored for VLSI Implementation", IEEE Trans. on NN, vol. 5, pp. 784-791, 1994.
[S&F94]   Shibata T. and Fukuda, T., "Hierarchical Intelligent Control for Robotic Motion", IEEE Trans. on NN, vol. 5, pp. 823-832, 1994.
[Vit94]   Vittoz, E., "Fundaments of Analog Design of Neural Networks", (a tutorial speech), 4th International Conference on Microelectronics for Neural Networks and Fuzzy Systems, Torino, Italy, 1994.
[Xil98]   XILINX Inc., "The Programmable Gate Array Data Book", 1998.
[E93 I]   Economou, G. - P. K., Nikolaidis, S. S., Metafas, D. E., and Goutis, C. E., "Development of a Technology Independent Library", J. of Microprocessing and Microprogramming, vol. 39, pp. 241-244, 1993.
[E94 I]   Economou, G. - P. K., Mariatos, E. P., Economopoulos, N. M., Lymberopoulos, D., and Goutis, C. E., "FPGA Implementation of Artificial Neural Networks: An Application on Medical Expert Systems", Proc. of 4th International Conference on Microelectronics for Neural Networks and Fuzzy Systems, pp. 287-293, Torino, Italy, Sep. 1994.
[E95]   Economou, G. - P., K., Hallas, J. A., Mariatos, E. P., and Goutis, C. E., "Artificial Neural Networks in Medical Decision Making Systems: An Application to Pulmonary Diseases' Diagnosis through VHDL Synthesis", Proc. of 1995 European Design and Test Conference & EuroASIC Exhibition, Paris, France, Mar. 1995.

6th Chapter

Merging the DSS into a Tele-Working Platform

"... and in consequence, are something of a mutual fit."
William James

6.1 Introduction

Tele-Working has been trying to ascertain itself as a dynamic means to enhance human productivity and resources, facilitate industry, and exploit modern technology facilities for more than a decade [Cro96]. It addresses a main cooperative work problem and the electronic data exchange between major public or private organizations and geographically distant users, free lancers, or regular employees. Currently, it is the cornerstone of a number of successful corporations on a global scale, either providing or utilizing new technologies. Some predictions state that its future lies with "trusted third parties" that combine data management and public key infrastructure, ready to offer enhanced message switching and translation in response to market trends.

Our Tele-Working Platform (TWP) was designed to cover the needs of MDs, thus forming an integrated Tele-Medicine Service (TMS). As a result, the new service was developed [E01] so as to fulfil a number of requirements: set-up a closed (but not restricted) collaborating group of MDs; provide extended real time audio/video/data communication; supply internet-like characteristics in a data secure environment; guarantee high quality of service. All the above issues had also to take care of fast vs. fair-cost connections.

Consequently, by its specifications, the TMS ought to offer:
- **Access Security**. No unauthorized admission is permitted to the service.
- **Performance**. Special attention was given to achieve small access/response times, so as to augment MDs/patients faith in the utilisation of the new technology.
- **Capacity**. The TWP can handle large numbers of simultaneous connections.
- **Multi-platform Architecture**. The TWP is strategically built to enact a Distributed Computing System (DCS) architecture thus permitting the exploitation of network resources (e.g. printers, file servers, etc.) while facing demanding task calls. Data, that are present within the distributed system, may be shared across all nodes of the TMS. This task-scheduling facet gives the platform flexibility, robustness, and potentially nearly limitless scalability.

The Tele-Working Platform has been developed so as to manage fault tolerance and enable non-stop availability. By making use of idle processing power within the distributed system, the overall efficiency can be increased by "load balancing" all the nodes. Synchronization across the TMS presents a management challenge that requires specialised technologies to be implemented; security enforcement can also be less than trivial to achieve.

6.2 Tele-Working Platform's General Characteristics

The goal was to build a TWP that would provide for 24-hour operational support, so that it would back-up a DCS and several joined service providers and networks. Its infrastructure should allow for adaptability to the customer's intranet, extranet, or other network requirement such as ISDN and/or ATM.

This DCS consists of a TWP addressing layer (TWPL) [Cro96], linking the communications facilities each host provides and the TMS application. TMS application consists of tools carrying out medical image processing, tele-conferencing, file record processing (both MDs' and patients' ones), various web-based applications, and our MDSS-based diagnosis. The TWPL acts like an in-between service amid program applications and networks, managing their disparate interaction across heterogeneous computing platforms. Fig. 6.1 represents the Tele-Working Platform services.

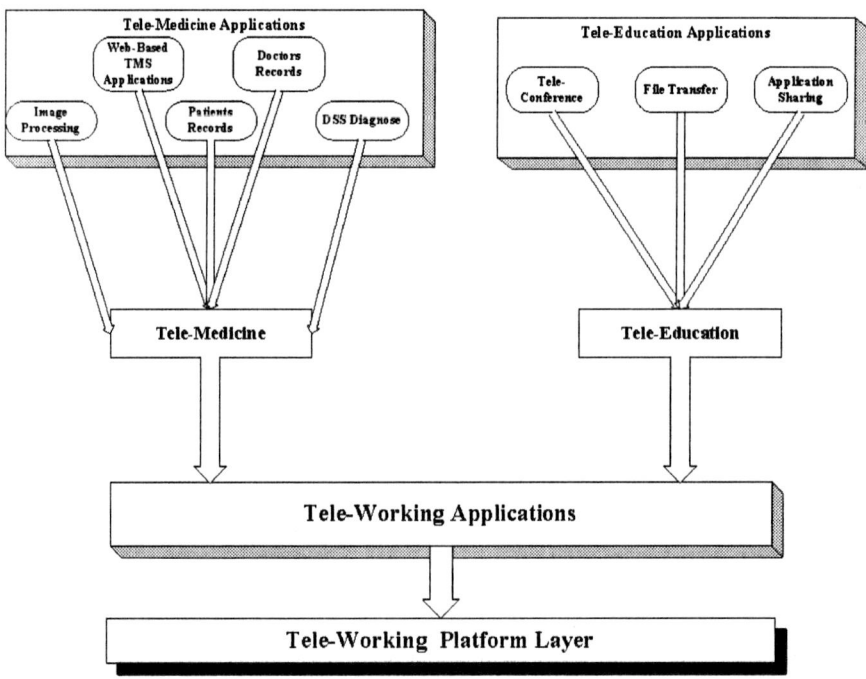

Figure 6.1: Tele-Medicine Service Schematic Representation

Those services are (TWPL components are given between parentheses):
- Patients' Records handling (input/process/store (multimedia) medical data).
- Message management (compose/send; deliver/read/store; reply to).
- Patients' Records Forwarding to another MD (waiting lists; distribution lists; automatic procedures for delivery, error correction, reading/processing).
- Clinic facilities operational time-scheduling.
- Real-time conferencing (chat-like (in personal/public virtual rooms); tele-conference mode with on-line collaborative medical image processing tools).
- Patients' catalogue (for MDs).
- MDs' catalogue (for the TWP).
- MDs' data handling (insertion/modification/finding/storing/deleting).

The following target groups were selected as possible users:
- Remote/collaborative (tele-)working MDs.
- Medical information retrieving organizations.
- Tele-Education networks (in medicine).
- Health-care providers.
- Tele-Attendance conferences covering surgical operations.

6.3 Two-tier Tele-Medicine Architecture

Before examining the requirements of our selected n-tier TWP architecture, the pros and cons of a two-tier system are given. Fig. 6.2 shows the layout of a typical two-tier information system: each user has to acquire a direct connection to the server.

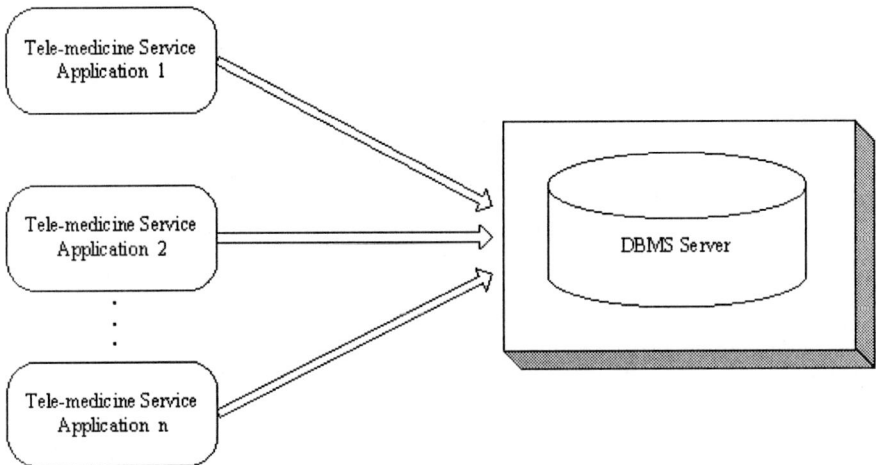

Figure 6.2: Two-tier Application and Direct User's Connection to the Server

Two-tier is currently the most common architecture [Del00] used for applications built on multi-user Database Management Systems (DBMS), such as Sun Oracle or MS-SQL Server. Each client's direct connection to the DBMS (or any application server) requires a vendor-specific library (i.e. an ODBC driver for MS-based operational systems). TMS client applications are typically required to log onto the DBMS independently and maintain an exclusive connection. The TMS client application is then responsible for preparing and sending SQL commands directly to the server (SQL is a programming language supporting data queries). The TMS client is also responsible for dealing with messages, errors, and streams of data returned by the database transaction manager engine.

The TMS client application commonly maintains some or all of the application's TMS logic. Whenever this changes, the TMS client application must be re-built and be re-distributed to all client TWPs. This can be a fairly tedious undertaking, and as a result, a fairly pressing demand has usually to be placed to justify the distribution of a new version of TWPL components.

The two-tier architecture of the TMS is at its best in an information system that employs a single data source. Unfortunately, the performance gains and centralization of the TMS logic within already-prepared SQL commands in the DBMS are usually unattainable when the system's data is spread across multiple servers [Vau98]. DBMSs usually have handy remote procedures stored, but this feature works only when every database server uses compatible DBMSs. In TMSs that utilize heterogeneous data sources, the two-tier architecture begins to quickly break down under the connections' number (as can be seen portrayed in Fig. 6.3).

Two-tier systems have been widely deployed in the industry, and consequently, the problems associated with them are very well known. Most problems arise under two circumstances: data being accessed by multiple client applications; system's data stored across multiple database servers.

Here's a summary of the two-tier TMS architecture problems:
- Changing TMS logic (database schema, data location, or connection information) requires the re-building of TMS client applications.
- Re-building those applications requires costly redistribution to client TWP.
- Database drivers must be installed and configured on each client TWP.
- Centralized TMS logic must be written in SQL stored procedures.
- Multiple DBMSs makes it difficult to maintain stored procedures.

6.4 Transition From Two-tier to n-tier Architecture

The aforementioned problems of the two-tier architecture were solved by the addition of an intermediate layer [Loc94]. The input of a set of TWPL components can serve to decouple client applications from data access code (Fig. 6.4).

Middle TWPL components are like stored procedures in that they allow to centralize a client's *mode d'employs* and re-use it across several applications. Unlike stored procedures, those components make it easy to access data across several DBMSs - even when of heterogeneous formats. Moreover, they can be written in programming languages such as MS-Visual Basic, MS-Visual C++, and Java, that offer many advantages in forwarding the same logic of SQL commands.

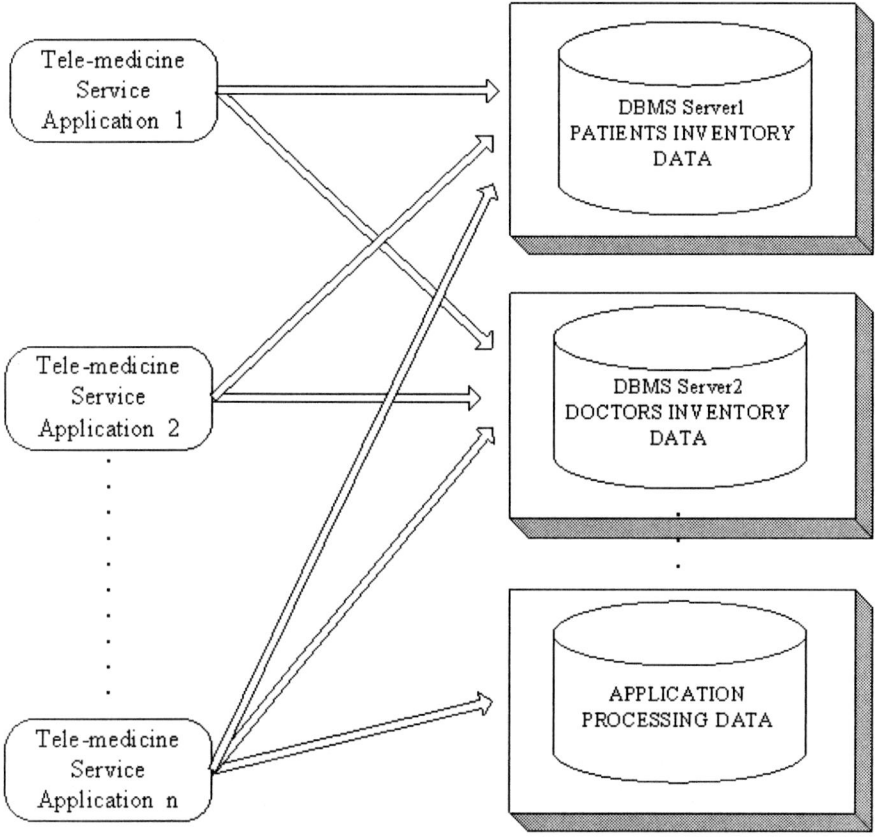

Figure 6.3: Two-tier Connections and Heterogeneous Data Sources

These components ensure a high degree of independence between the underlying systems (DBMSs, www Servers, Application Servers, etc.) and the TMS applications. They are used to transfer information from one client application to one or more other applications or clients, shielding the application *per se* from dependencies inherent in communications protocols, operating systems, and hardware platforms. Generally, this TWPL provides a set of services specifically geared towards supporting DCS. The services ensure that TWP is scalable, reliable, secure, and available for use and gives high performance. The introduction of this layer also eliminated connection costly dependencies between TWP client applications and multiple DBMSs up to 70%.

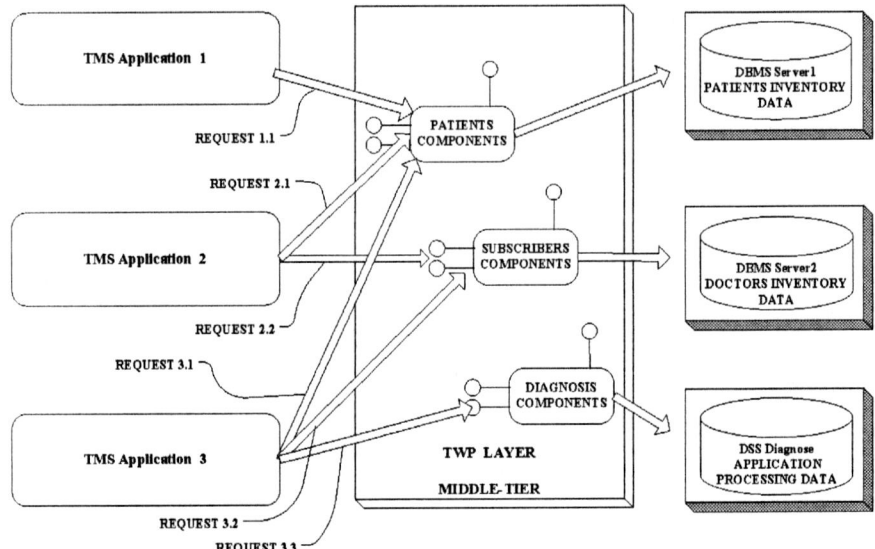

Figure 6.4: Introducing a Middle layer of TWP Components

TWPL components are employed by using the Component Object Model (COM) as their implementation basis [Ise00]. COM can serve as the basis for communications between the TMS client applications and the n-tier objects. As a result, TWP running the TMS client applications need only to be COM-aware, instead of having to rely on database drivers as they do in the two-tier model.

Another advantage is that COM allows an n-tier programmer to update the TWPL components without requiring a re-compilation and re-distribution of TMS client applications. Thus a TMS logic is easily changed. A TMS's data can change storage formats and new DBMSs can be brought on line with little effort. The necessary modifications are made in the middle tier, allowing TMS client applications to remain in unaltered operation. Fig. 6.5 presents the TWP layer.

6.5 Interface Implementation

In order for the TMS application to use TWPL components, a user-defined interface TWPL (I-TWPL) was created. The creation of several classes that implement the I-TWPL interface led to the plug-and-play benefits of the polymorph implementation. Different types of TWPL objects exhibit different behaviour, but they are all controlled through the same interface.

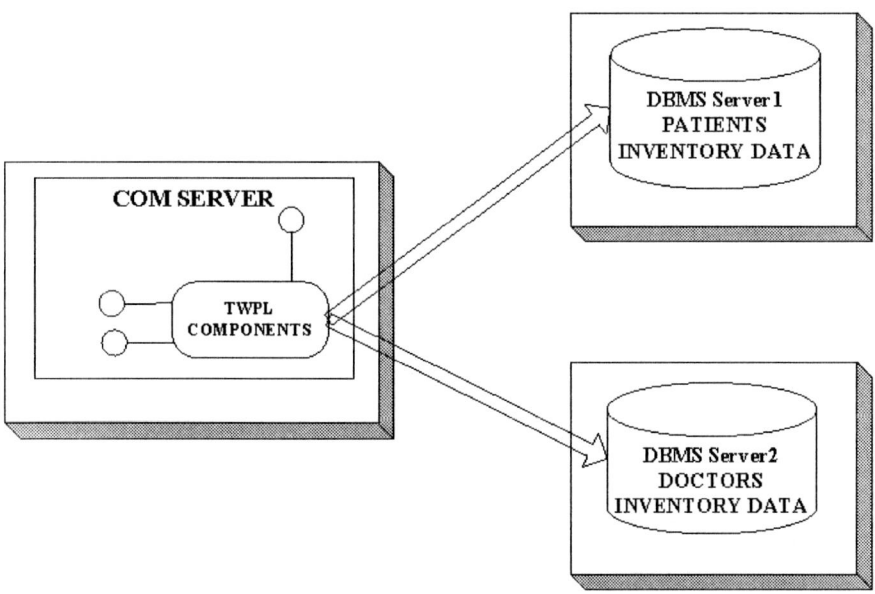

Figure 6.5: The Mapping between TWPL Components and Data Access layer

From a versioning point of view, this design permits the improvement of the behaviour of various TWPL components by introducing new interfaces into the application. Interfaces such as I-TWPL2, I-TWPL3, and ITWPL4 permit the safe extension of the behaviour of those components. The best part about this approach is that the revision of clients and components can be independently achieved. Older TMS clients and TWPL objects can use earlier interfaces, while newer TMS clients and TWPL objects are able to communicate through newer interfaces. All are made possible through the interface support run-time type inspection [Sta00].

6.6 TWPL COM Components' Features

User-defined interfaces are of great value in large applications, because they bestow the ability of code re-using, trouble-free maintaining, and operation non-stop expansion. COM follows these concepts of interface-based programming:
- Requires a formal separation of interface and implementation - that is, it requires that clients communicate with components exclusively through interface references. This ensures that clients never build dependencies on the classes that back-up components - that in turn allows COM programmers to revise their component code without worrying about breaking into client applications' one.

- COM clients are able to obtain run-time information type from components. A COM client can always query a component and ask whether it supports a specific interface. If the requested interface is not supported, the client finds it and gracefully degrades to the most suitable subsequent one.

The entire TMS application was written in a single programming language and the source code was compiled as a unique process. However, COM clients and COM components can be written in different languages and can run in different processes on different TWPs. COM is able to solve problems at the physical implementation level to achieve the benefits of interface-based programming.

6.6.1 TWPL Component v Table

When utilising COM, clients and components communicate through vTables [Ise00]. Thus TWPL components, as well as TMS clients, can heavily rely on the use of their internal TWP resources. In COM, clients bind to components at run time; however, to properly communicate with a TWPL component, a TMS application client must know a few things at compile time, mostly:
- The type of component it wants to create.
- The interface(s) it will use to communicate with the component.
- The calling syntax for each method in the interface(s).

6.6.2 Interface Definition Language and Globally Unique Identifiers

The language independence is achieved by COM trough providing a universal way for servers to make information known about the interfaces and the co-classes of components they contain. COM was standardized as a programming language called Interface Definition Language (IDL). IDL provides a way to define a set of interfaces and co-classes in a manner that is programming language-neutral. This means that any COM-capable language can be used to implement or use the definitions from an IDL source file. The IDL source file must be fed to an IDL compiler (e.g. MS-MIDL [Ise00]). MS-MIDL generates some source files used by the C/C++ programmers and a special binary database called a type library [Ise00].

A type library is a catalogue that describes interfaces, co-classes, and other resources in a server. Each interface is defined with a set of methods; each co-class is defined with one or more interfaces [Ise00].

6.7 TWPL Components Activation

The TMS application discovers the necessary co-class component as well as which interfaces it supports at compile time through the type library. However, COM requires that no other dependencies be built between clients and co-classes. This is why the TMS application uses a supported interface when it binds to and communicates with a TWPL component created from the co-class. This act of loading and binding to a component is called **activation**. The TMS application activates a TWPL component with some help from the COM library.

Activation support is built into COM's infrastructure because the TMS application is never allowed to create a TWPL component using a visible concrete class definition from the server. If this were the case, the TMS application would be required to see the class definition and know about the TWPL component's data layout at compile time. Instead, COM puts the responsibility of creating the TWPL component on the server that holds the co-class definition. The infrastructure support supplied by COM plays the role of a middleman. It takes an activation request from the TMS application and forwards it to the server. The COM component that assists activation is the Service Control Manager (SCM) [Ros93].

When the TMS application processes a certain co-class's identification, the SCM uses configuration information to locate the particular resource server. This means that a COM server requires an associated physical path to its location. When the TMS application calls a co-class, the following happen:
- The TWP libraries (resident programming software) forward to the SCM the requested co-class's (unique) authentication data.
- The SCM locates the particular resource server (loading its code if necessary).
- The server creates the component authentication of the type specified.
- The server returns an interface reference of the type specified to the SCM.
- The SCM forwards the interface reference back to the client.
- The TMS client is bound to the TWPL component.
- The SCM is no longer needed and therefore drops out of use.
- The TMS client invokes methods on the TWPL component.

In conclusion, the SCM is really just a matchmaker. Yet, for this architecture to work properly, the SCM must have a predefined way of interacting with the server. The COM server must therefore provide support for the TWPL component activation through which the SCM can make activation requests.

6.7.1 Class Factories
Server-side activation rules are defined in the COM specifications [Vau98]. COM uses a common software technique known as the factory pattern, in which the code that actually creates the TWPL component is contained in the same file. This eliminates the need for the TMS application or the SCM to know about the class definition behind the TWPL component being created. The key advantage of this technique is that it allows class authors to revise their code without worrying about TMS application dependencies, such as a TWPL component's data layout.

Every COM server must provide class factories for the SCM. After the TMS application is bound to a TWPL component, the SCM is no longer needed. At this point, the TWPL component must provide a certain base level of functionality to the TMS application. In addition to implementing each method in every supported interface, a TWPL component must manage its own lifetime and allow TMS applications to move back and forth between the various interfaces it supports.

6.7.2 The IUnknown Interface
COM has one interface from which all other interfaces derive: IUnknown. Every interface must derive directly from it or from an interface that has it at the root of its inheritance chain. IUnknown is at the top of every COM interface hierarchy.

IUnknown expresses the base behaviour of a COM component (TWPL component) as opposed to a domain-specific one being experienced through a user-defined interface. IUnknown allows every TWPL component to manage its own lifetime. It also allows the TMS application to query a TWPL component

With the reference counting scheme employed by COM, multiple clients can connect to a TWPL component. If a TMS client application never explicitly deletes a TWPL component, it is impossible for a TMS client application to delete a component that is currently being used by another client.

6.7.3 Binding Technique
vTable binding is always best. It is faster than the other two kinds by an order of magnitude. vTable are always used bindings as long as the following are true:
- The client project contains a reference to the type library.
- The reference is forwarded to the deafault interface or a creatable class.
- The component exposes vTables for dual/pure vTable interfaces.

6.7.4 Out-Of-Process Server
COM makes remote communication possible with a pair of help components called the proxy and the stub. Figure 6.6 shows how the proxy and the stub are employed. The proxy runs in the TMS's application process, while the stub runs in the TWPL component's process. Proxy and stub establish a communication channel using Remote Procedure Calls (RPCs) as the inter-process mechanism.

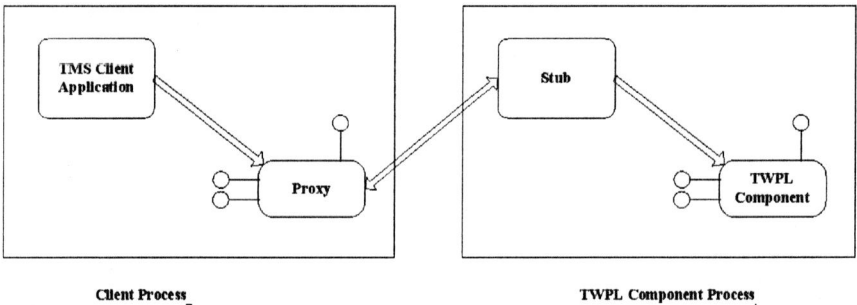

Figure 6.6: A Proxy/Stub layer

The communication channel passes data back and forth during remote method execution. This act of serializing method parameters for transmission through the proxy/stub architecture is known as **marshalling**.

When the TMS application invokes a method on the proxy, the proxy forwards the request to the stub. To properly transmit this request, the proxy must marshal the method's inbound parameters to the stub. When the stub receives the request, it un-marshals the inbound parameters and locally performs the call on the TWPL component. After the TWPL component has completed the method, the stub prepares a response packet that includes outbound parameters and a return value.

The data is then marshalled back to the proxy. The proxy un-marshals the data in the response packet and returns control back to the client.

The best part about this remote architecture is that neither the TMS application nor the TWPL component "realize" that each of the other is remote. The TMS application "considers" the proxy as the TWPL component; the latter, on the other hand, that the stub is the TMS application. This allows COM programmers to write code for both clients and components without regards to whether the components will be activated from an in-process server or an out-of-process server. This powerful feature is known as **location transparency**.

There is a proxy/stub pair for each connected interface. This allows a TMS client and a TWPL component to have two or more proxy/stub pairs connecting them at once. It makes sense that the proxy/stub pair is associated with the interface because the interface describes the methods that need to be remote. With an interface definition stored in a type library, COM can determine the exact manner in which the data should be marshalled to the component and back. This is why IDL allows the specification parameters such as [in], [out], and [in, out].

The proxy and the stub have their work cut out for them. They must work together to give both the TMS application and the TWPL component the perception that they are running in a single process on a single thread. They create this illusion by constructing a call stack in the TWPL component's process that is identical to the one in the TMS's process. Any data sitting on the call stack in the TMS's process must be marshalled to the component's process. The stub is responsible for un-marshalling all the data and setting up the call stack, which might include pointers to data that does not "live" on the stack.

COM provides a system service called the **universal marshal** that automatically builds the proxy/stub code at run time. It does this by examining interface definitions in a type library. When an interface reference is exported from the component's process, the universal marshal builds and loads a stub component. When the interface reference is imported into a client process, the universal marshal creates a proxy and binds it to the client. The communication channel that is established between the proxy and the stub can thus remote method requests between the TMS application and the TWPL component.

6.7.5 Out-of-Process Activation

The SCM must acquire a reference to a class factory component in every activation request, but this occurs in quite a different way when the server runs in its own process. With an in-process server, the SCM connects to a class factory component through a well-known component authentication.

When an out-of-process server is launched, it must register a class factory TWPL component for each of its creatable co-classes with the COM library. The SCM maintains a machine-wide internal table called the class table, which holds the class factory component references for every registered co-class's authentications. The SCM can scan through this table and retrieve a reference to any local class factory component that has been registered.

When the SCM receives an activation request for a co-class that is implemented in a local server, it looks through the class table to determine whether it has already been registered. If it is found in the class table, the server is up and running. If it has not been registered, the SCM launches the server process and waits so that the server can be registered. After that, the SCM can revisit the class table and acquire the needed reference to the class factory component. Then, it asks the server to create an instance in a manner similar to the in-process scenario.

After the SCM creates the out-of-process component, it must bind the TWPL component to the TMS applications using a proxy/stub pair. When the TWPL component exports an interface reference to the SCM, the SCM calls on the universal marshal to create the stub component; then it calls on the universal marshal to create a proxy one to bind the application and the component together.

When the local SCM determines that the component authentication in an activation request resides on a different TWP, it searches across the network and establishes a connection with a remote SCM. Inter-host communication requires that the activation request be passed through an authentication/authorization layer. The remote SCM goes through the same activation process described above.

The only real change is that the interface reference must be marshalled from one TWP to another. The interface reference is exported from the remote server process in the same manner as for a local one. When the interface reference is unmarshalled into the client process, the proxy is populated with enough information to get back to a specific stub for a specific component on a specific host.

6.7.6 Location Transparency Importance
This process of binding a remote TWPL component sounds complicated, but the SCM takes care of it. A TMS application does not have to concern itself with the details of in-process activation vs. out-of-process activation. The TMS application requests a specific component authentication and is then bound to the TWPL one. After the binding takes place, the TMS application goes about its business by invoking methods and accessing properties. The TMS application perceives that the TWPL component is close by, but that does not have to be the case.

In the out-of-process scenario, the TWPL component also perceives that the client is in the same process. This means that the details of in-process vs. out-of-process activation are hidden from TWPL component code as well as the TMS client application. The ability of programmers to write client code and component code for an in-process relationship and have the code work automatically across process boundaries is one of the most powerful features of COM.

Figure 6.7 shows 3 different ways of server employment without changing any code for the TMS application or the TWPL component.

COM's ability to seamlessly combine remote components is known as **location transparency**. It also means that components can be redeployed around the network with little impact on code (and only when first-written).

6.8 Internet-based Tele-Medicine Service Applications
Two of the selected target groups (§6.2) are information retrieving activities and Tele-Education networks (in medicine). The needs of the MDs to be continuously

informed of Medical Science achievements and their patients' health condition, enforced the introduction of Internet Information Servers (IIS) in the TMS.

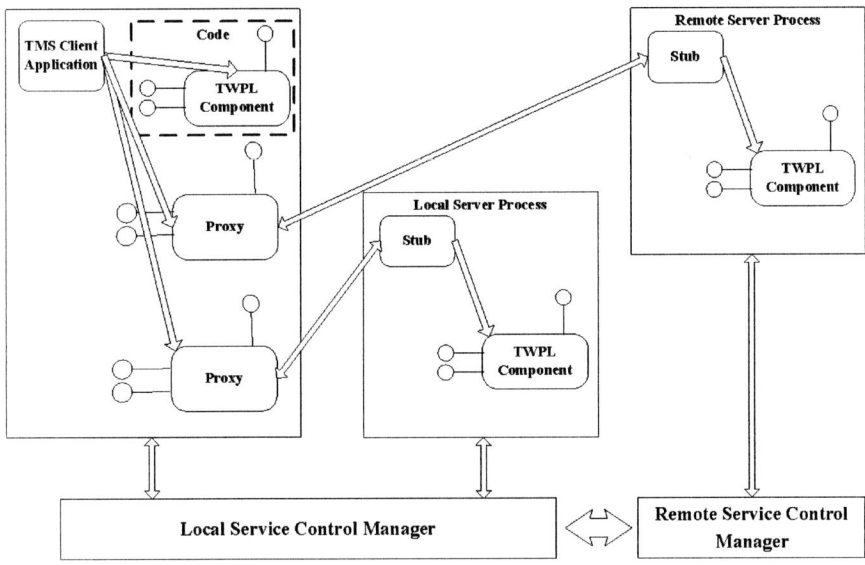

Figure 6.7: Inter-process Communication

Internet technologies have been utilized wherever possible. HTML [Mor02] and XML [Wyk02] are currently the best way to create a cross-platform IIS application. Also, applications built around a standard Web browser significantly reduce TWP configuration and employment costs. Finally, Web-based systems can be used to reach a much larger audience than is possible with typical LAN/WAN-based architecture. The end-user interface of the TMS is thus a combination of static and dynamic HTML pages. XML documents containing the actual data are being parsed and displayed on the MD's web browser. MDs have access to up-to-date information about their patients' progress and Medical Science developments.

The system was designed and implemented as a distributed service with a central point of access: the TWPL. The distributed nature of the system complies with the MDs' requirement to keep under their control all the information for their patients' and integrate their existing infrastructure with the new TMS applications.

The TWPL components act like a medical device index with essential information for each patient and medicine's achievements, conference proceedings etc., which allows the MD to perform first filtering of the available results according to their queries and then focus to those that better satisfies his requirements. The main components of the web-based TMS are (Fig. 6.8):
- Oracle 9i RDBMS [Pri01].

128

- MS-SQL 2000 DBMS [Del00].
- End-User Interface (XML, HTML).
- DCOM mechanism (MS-based COM programming environment) [DCOM].
- Additional services [E01], [Sot02].

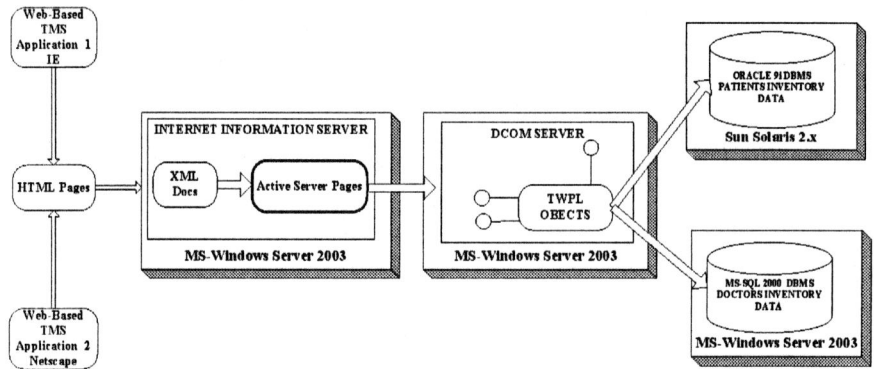

Figure 6.8: TWPL, IIS, and HTML

MDs access the Patients and Doctors Inventory Data through an HTML interface, which consists of both static and dynamic contents:
- The dynamic HTML pages are produced by stored procedures in the Oracle 9i RDBMS and MS-SQL/.NET DBMS. These stored procedures produce XML files that are parsed and displayed by JavaScript [Goo01] that runs inside static HTML pages on the browser side (i.e., MS-Internet Explorer, Netscape Navigator, etc.).
- The static HTML pages and the additional files that they use are stored in a directory structure on the server machines that hosts the Oracle 9i RDBMS, MS-SQL .NET DBMS and the Internet Information Server (IIS).
- XML files are used extensively for data presentation [Wyk02].

The IIS provides the environment for the Active Server Pages (ASP) [Kot02]. Both static and dynamic HTML content are mixed to provide the user interface. The static HTML pages provide the basic structure of the interface containing navigation buttons, links, etc. They also contain JavaScript code that interprets (parses) the dynamically produced XML pages and display the results.

The dynamic content is created when the end-user requests pass through the IIS to stored procedures in the Oracle 9i RDBMS and MS-SQL .NET DBMS. The stored procedures access the data in the databases and they produce XML or HTML output that is fed back to the browser. The extensive use of XML

documents is made for data presentation. The XML data are parsed on the browser side in two ways, depending on the browser:
- For MS-Internet Explorer the embedded XML Parser has been used.
- For Netscape Navigator a custom Java Applet that encapsulates the SUN Java XML Parser has been developed to ensure user accessibility.

6.9 Conclusion

The team's desire to build the Tele-Working Platform for Tele-Medicine Service was the many applications to implement it in a flexible, user friendly, foolproof, fruitful, and most convenient manner. It seeks to convey unexploited resources and to combine high-end technological solutions, especially in rural, remote regions where no other MDs collaboration means is available. At the same time, its structures were made to rely on implementation software facets that would assure its scalability.

Attributes of the platform and service, such as its adaptability and promptness to satisfy many work demands, are going to be enhanced by future Tele-Centres. Their use will be to combine the many, disparate small networks of the main TWP.

6.10 References

[Ros93] Rosenberry, W. and Teague, J., "Distributing Applications across DCE and Windows NT", O'Reilly, 1993.
[Loc94] Lockhart, H. W., "OSF DCE, Guide to Developing Distributed Applications", McGraw-Hill, 1994.
[Cro96] Crowcroft, J., "Open Distributed Systems", UCL, 1996.
[Vau98] Vaughn, W. R., "Hitchhiker's Guide to Visual Basic® and SQL Server™", Microsoft Press, 1998.
[Del00] Delaney, K., "Inside Microsoft® SQL Server™ 2000", Microsoft Press, 2000.
[Ise00] Iseminger, C., "COM+ Developer's Reference Library", Microsoft Press, 2000.
[Sta00] Stamatakis, W., "Design Patterns: elements of reusable object-oriented software", Microsoft Press, 2000.
[Goo01] Goodman, D., "JavaScript Bible", Wiley, 2001.
[Pri01] Price, J., "Oracle 9i JDBC Programming", Oracle Press, 2001.
[Kot02] Kothari, N. and Datye, V., "Developing Microsoft® ASP.NET Server Controls and Components", Microsoft Press, 2002.
[Mor02] Morrison, M., "Faster Smarter HTML & XML", Microsoft Press, 2002.
[Sot02] Sotiriades P., Economou, G. - P., and Lymberopoulos, D., "Enhanced Applications of an ISDN-based Tele-Working Platform", IASTED International Conference Communication Systems and Networks (CSN 2002), pp. 384-391, September 9-12, 2002 Malaga, Spain.
[Wyk02] Wyke, R. A., Rehman, S., and Leupen, B., "XML Programming (Core Reference)", Microsoft Press, 2002.
[DCOM] DCOM, http://www.microsoft.com.

[E01] Economou, G. - P. K., Karavatselou, E., Chassomeris, C., and Lymberopoulos, D., "A Novel Tele-Medicine System", On-line Symposium for Electronic Engineers, http://www.osee.NET/pro_bio_systems.html.

7th Chapter

Conclusions - Future Work

All that we are is the result of what we have thought:
it is founded on our thought, it is made up of our thoughts
I. J. Dhammapada

7.1 Conclusions

A new decision support system with modular structure is proposed. It is applied in areas where the human experience constitutes the most important factor for the decisions' promotion and it is configured on a basis of artificial neural networks. The ANNs provide it with the ability to be productively adapted to the applications' structures it approaches, exploit the grouping of input data that the expert handles, and process them in the System hierarchical stages.

The ANNs exploitation in all the stages of the System's Layers constitutes an innovation of the whole project. Previous Systems used to assign the Networks classifying functions, pattern recognition tasks, or quick processing of input data, implementing additional inference engines. ANNs in the aforementioned DSS comply with all the above roles; moreover they are used to back-up a decision.

The taught System is input data, this would promote the feeding of new ones, processes them, concludes to intermediate decisions, and ultimately provides the final one. Occasionally, time has to elapse so promoted inputs. Therefore, it has been modelled so that possible input changes are taken into consideration in case of their temporal evolution.

When compared to previous DSSs, the proposed System is not based on: pre-processing or the symbolic representation of input data; the creation of a knowledge base and its control techniques; and the achievement of the appropriate inference engines. Therefore, its memory demands are much less. The ANNs constitute the System processing cells by means of which the application structures are implemented. Networks successions materialize the System's hierarchical operation from the input to the output stage, they are arranged depending on the application, and through their interconnections the transition of the intermediate outputs to next inputs is performed. The generalization of the System's Learning Patterns into new inputs is based on ANNs robust inherent characteristics.

The System's modular architecture and its ANNs, give the ability to its user to exploit all intermediate decisions (ANNs responds). Also, while the System runs through its operation flow, it follows the application's structures and the standardization of its performance heads towards the final decision.

Extended experiments took place so that the Network on which the System would be based was chosen. The experiments focused on their implementation, teaching, and generalization accuracy facets. As a consequence, the FFA-ANN was promoted as the basic unit and the application of Kalman's equations on the back propagation rule during their learning.

The FFA-ANN showed learning easiness, undemanding expansion of its inputs and Synapses to handle new data and different architectures, and good convergence speed of its outputs into the chosen Patterns. Moreover, the learning was made through 2 learning algorithms: back propagation rule and the application of Kalman's equations. Only a hidden Slab [§1.2] was sufficient for their learning, keeping the number of the hidden Neurons very small.

The System was applied to all pulmonary and haematology diseases separately, reaching very good performances. The ANNs were taught with the experience of MDs' teams and the patients' clinical data, and were tested extensively during their generalization into new inputs. The coverage of all the diseases of each medical region constitutes another innovation of the whole project. Other Medical Systems only considered a few diseases, covered some sections of human organs, even utilized other means to ensure ANNs' results.

Because of the evolutionary nature of medical data, the patients' clinical data are not always recorded with the same completeness and are therefore often incomplete - useless for ANNs learning. This problem was faced through a new form of Learning Patterns mapping. The proposed new form is not restricted to the medical field only but can also be used for the learning of more general ANNs.

The new mapping form inserts each input data component separately into the Networks. Furthermore, it gives a different evaluation value to each one and adds a number of pseudo inputs in the Patterns to better balance the ANNs' output classes. Consequently, incomplete medical data are also fed to the System and the pseudo inputs complete with balancing components the Learning Patterns in order for the total number of the contributed ones to be kept constant for each output. Experimental learning with the new form components has proven the better operation of the Networks. Previous research efforts did not use incomplete data or they used to statistically complete them (according to generally accepted principles).

Furthermore, the FFA-ANNs convergence engine to their Learning Patterns was also studied. The use of smaller numbers of hidden Neurons is proposed from what the bibliography suggests. The Neurons can increase in slow rates, preserving the previous teaching's Weights and so averting the re-initialisation of the Network. The Synapses Weights' configurations are topologically analysed and their handling is correspondingly proposed. The analysis of these FFA-ANN elements (e.g. the number of hidden Neurons) results in "rules of the thumb" for intervening on them and mainly decrease their implementation hardware.

An architecture for the implementation of the new System in hardware is suggested next. Artificial neuron operations from digital circuits is proposed, by implementing a multiplier-adder/accumulator, an approximation of the Sigmoid function, and the numerical accuracy strict definition. FPGAs are first used to exploit the re-targeting capability they offer.

The structure for the MDSS implementation in hardware is then developed by means of utilizing the environment of the hardware description language VHDL. Design independence is ensured, along to the other benefits of hardware.

Finally, the merging of the proposed MDSS into a Tele-Working Platform was performed. The resulting TMS was more generally set-up and all the necessary configuration steps were given to satisfy large remote collaboration schemes.

7.2 Future Work

Our primary aim was to apply the System to other fields of medicine, with the ultimate purpose of producing an MDMS that will be able to analyse in full a patient's condition for many other diseases. Already, preliminary research is pointing to the field of otorhinolaryngology [Pap02].

Moreover, the expansion of input data gives a valid direction to the system, as geographically restricted data could limit its proper operation. On the other hand, the supply of input data from other hospitals or MD teams could probably increase the number of the MDSS's inputs as MDs probably would belong to other "schools". Therefore, the exploitation of the System can be achieved only through its thorough use in new patient cases - that would demonstrate new symptom grouping [Nag01].

The example of the Pulmonary team emphasises the use of the Medical System for identifying fatal diseases such as tuberculosis or lung cancer. This specialization will not limit the central MDSS's operation flow to which it also be integrated, but it is hoped to be able to promote properly the existence or non-existence of the diseases in (very) early stages [Leo02].

New topologies and ANNs' teaching algorithms could also be used in the medical decision support system. The fact that the linear approaches of FFA-ANNs gave adequate performances when compared to their software counterparts, could prompt for their functionality in more complicated applications [Teo99].

The utilized artificial neurons on which FFA-ANNs are based, were always the same in structure. Therefore, the use of specialized Neurons in a hierarchical structure, and an appropriate learning algorithm would probably ameliorate the System's effectiveness or would limit its demands in hardware.

The System uses as inputs data that are also requested by its operation flow [Bro00] and that are demanded for its further processing. Those data are mainly laboratory records though they could be composed of other measurements, etc. Some of the latter data could be integrated in the MDSS operation (e.g. medical image processing based on ANNs).

The wiping out of whatever redundancy in its interconnections, that the proposed decision support system can present, is another high priority target. The number of the artificial neural networks, the artificial neurons, and their synapses need detailed analysis for the verification of their offer to the whole System. This will be achieved through the use of the Medical System in large scale so its most important units, that characterize its function, are distinguished. Another starting point could be the standardization of the "rules of the thumb" developed for learning (mainly intervening in Weights and the new Patterns' mapping form).

Other areas where the human experience has a decisive role in the decision making procedure could be new implementation areas. Diagnostic systems, controlling of procedures, observation of the economic assets are some of the applications that are characterized by structures and hierarchical processing of their inputs. The adaptation of the decision support system to these areas or the redesigning of its structure so as to approach application structures of a different type will confirm its generalization aim and will define a System for an extended use.

7.3 References

[Teo99] Teodorescu, H.-N. L., Kandel, A., and Jain, L., "Fuzzy and Neuro-Fuzzy Systems in Medicine", CRC Press, 1999.

[Bro00] Bronzino, J. D., "The Biomedical Engineering Handbook", CRC Press, 2000.

[Nag01] Naguib, R. N. G. and Sherbet G. V., "Artificial Neural Networks in Cancer Diagnosis, Prognosis, and Patient Management", CRC Press, 2001.

[Leo02] Leondes, C. T., "Computational Methods in Biophysics, Biomaterials, Biotechnology, and Medical Systems", Kluwer Academic Publishers, 2002.

[Pap02] Papadas, T., Charokopos, N., Karamouzis, M. V., Pierakeas, C., Symeonidi, M., Economou, G. - P. K., and Goumas, P., "Rehabilitation after Laryngectomy: A Practical Approach and Guidelines for Patients", Journal of Cancer Education, vol. 17, pp. 37 - 39, 2002.

Appendix I

The MDSS Demo
Why think when you can simulate?
J. A. Anderson and Ed. Rosenfeld

Application

The MDSS software application was compiled into a demo program that demonstrates a great deal of the full System's traits. This program, as well instruction notes and other material, can be reached by the following web page:

http://www.wcl.ee.upatras.gr/prj/gpe/web_p0.html

Next figures picture this demo's medical processing flow:

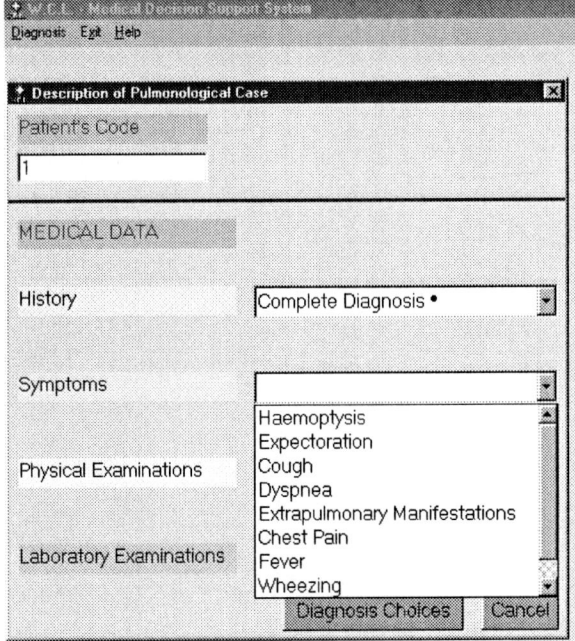

Figure I.1:MDSSs' Initial Medical Data Input Screen

Basically, upon "clicking" on the *Diagnosis* option Fig. I.1 appears. The user is then prompted to insert the *Patients' Code* and start feeding medical data by making appropriate selections on each *History*'s, *Symptoms*', *Physical Examinations*', or *Laboratory Examinations*' "combo box" (a visual programming component capable to provide user-friendly selections).

Should a user select a symptom, a screen similar to Fig. I.2 appears:

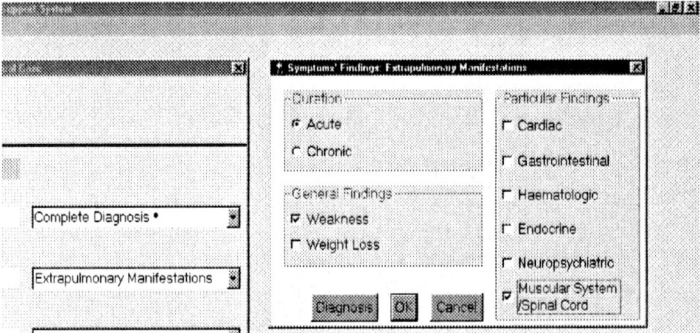

Figure I.2: Inputs for a Symptom's Sub-category

"Radio Buttons" or "Check Boxes" can be utilized to input medical data. Once finished, by clicking the *Diagnosis* button, a screen similar to Fig. I.3 appears:

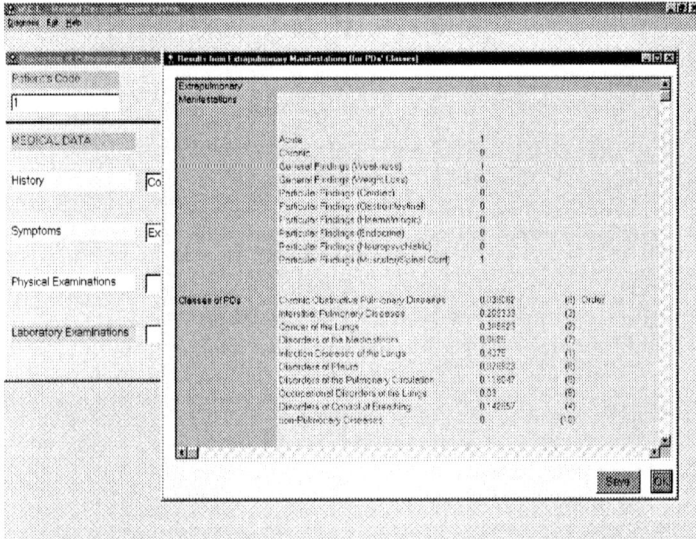

Figure I.3: A Sub-diagnosis Resulted from Fig. I.2's Inputs

At this point, a user could save or discard these results. However, he/she could also save them and choose not to use them later on, thus building diagnosis scenarios. Fig. I.4 shows a diagnosis screen:

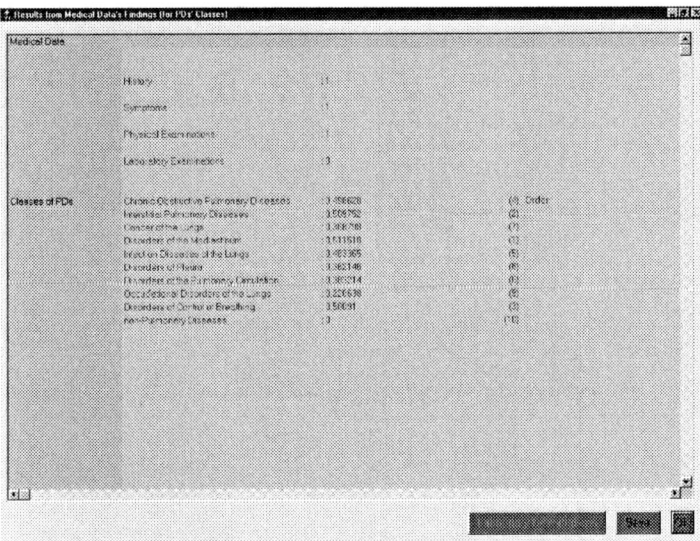

Figure I.4: A Final Diagnosis Screen

An output class of a disease is an active entry that can be clicked to show suggested laboratory examinations for this entry. Fig. I.5 shows possible ones:

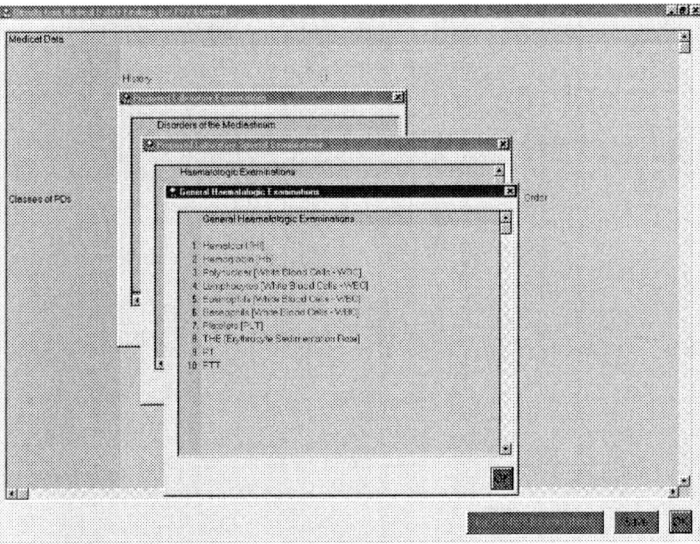

Figure I.5: Suggested Laboratory Examinations Screens

Appendix II

More on Type Libraries
It made engineering sense
H. Schildt

GUIDs
Type library files have many possible extensions, including .tlb, .dll, .exe, .olb, and .ocx. COM co-classes and interfaces are identified by a globally unique identifier (GUID), which is a 128-bit integer. Most compilers and databases do not support 128-bit integers, so GUIDs are usually stored in other formats. Solutions are:
- A data structure representation by means of a set of smaller integral values.
- A 32-character hexadecimal of GUID expression form that makes it readable. This string format is also used to store GUIDs in the MS-Windows registry.

The TWPL COM library supplies a function named CoCreateGUID, which is used to generate a new GUID. The function relies on an algorithm that uses information such as the unique identifier from the computer's network card and system clock to create a GUID that is guaranteed to be unique across time and space. This allows to cut-and-paste GUIDs into IDL and C++ source code.

Each COM of TWPL interface has an associated GUID called an interface ID (IID). Each co-class has an associated GUID called a class ID (CLSID). When examining an IDL, each interface and co-class show a Universally Unique Identifier (UUID) attribute. UUIDs and GUIDs are the same thing.

These CLSIDs and IIDs are compiled into a server's type library. A GUID becomes the physical name for an interface or a co-class. When a client application is compiled against the type library, these GUIDs are also compiled into the client's binary image. This enables the client application to ask for a specific co-class and interface whenever it needs to create and bind to an object.

Appendix III

COM/CORBA/XML & HTML

Enough research will tend to support your project
Murphy's Law of Research

COM

COM defines how components and their clients interact. In COM threading, there are primarily two entities: the components, and the COM apartment that hosts these components. The components are developed to run in certain types of apartments and have a corresponding threading model value in the registry to reflect the type of apartment in which they can run. The second entity, the COM apartment, hosts these components. The aforementioned interaction is defined such that the client and the component can connect without the need of any intermediary system component. Microsoft's distributed COM (DCOM) extends the protocol to support communication among objects on different computers on a LAN, a WAN, or even the Internet. The advantages that DCOM offers are:
- Location independence.
- Performance.
- Load balancing.
- Protocol neutrality.
- Connection management.
- Bandwidth and latency.
- Fault tolerance.
- Platform neutrality.
- Scalability.
- Security.
- Ease of deployment.
- Integration with otherInternet protocols

CORBA

The Common Object Request Broker Architecture (CORBA) is the Object Management Group's answer to the need for interoperability among the rapidly proliferating number of hardware and software products available today. Simply stated, CORBA allows applications to communicate with one another no matter where they are located or who has designed them. CORBA 1.1 was introduced in 1991 by Object Management Group (OMG) and defined the Interface Definition Language (IDL) and the Application Programming Interfaces (API) that enable client/server object interaction within a specific implementation of an Object Request Broker (ORB). CORBA 2.0, adopted in December of 1994, defines true interoperability by specifying how ORBs from different vendors can interoperate.

CORBA is a competing standard for both COM/DCOM. It defines an abstract object model that describes components and their interfaces. It also provides standard mappings from the abstract object definition to concrete programming languages, but it does not define a binary standard in any way. Different implementations that adhere to this standard can achieve, at the most, source level compatibility, but not inter-changeability of binary components.

CORBA also defines a standard for inter- Object Request Broker (ORB) communication that allows 2 compliant ORB implementations to invoke methods on objects on each other's machine. Again, it defines a separate inter-ORB communication protocol called IIOP, which is targeted for use on the Internet. It accommodates the intersection of all inter-ORB protocols.

XML & HTML

Extensible Mark-up Language, or XML as it is more commonly known, is more than just the latest trend or TLA (Three-Letter Acronym). XML is paving the way to the next generation of the World Wide Web: the Information Marketplace1. Most importantly, this technology is being implemented today, in Internet-time. Since the release of the XML 1.0 Specification2 in early February 1998, some of the most influential companies in the technology industry have announced their support of this standard. While HTML existed without even a specification from 1991 until 1996, XML has emerged practically overnight, requiring developers to come up to speed quickly. This Primer teaches the basics of XML and answers some of the fundamental questions about XML technology.

XML is defined by the World Wide Web Consortium (W3C) as "...the universal format for structured documents and data on the Web". On the other hand, Hyper Text Mark-up Language (HTML) is described by the W3C as "the lingua franca for publishing hypertext on the World Wide Web". Both XML and HTML are subsets of the Standard Generalized Markup Language (SGML). Since XML and HTML have the same parent, they share similarities:

- Both are "mark-up languages" that use tags and attributes to described data.
- Both are text-based, meaning that the minimum you need to view or to create them is a text editor (like MS-Notepad). The fact that they are text-based also indicates that they work well with current protocols, such as HTTP.
- Both XML and HTML use a Document Type Definition (DTD). Think of the DTD as a document that describes the structure of another document. With respect to HTML, the DTDs are published and managed by the W3C. The differences between HTML versions 2.0, 3.2, and 4.01 are captured in that version's DTD. The DTD for HTML version 3.2 extends the DTD for HTML 2.0 allowing the use of new tags and attributes. The key here is these DTDs are set by the W3C and cannot be extended by the Web developer. This isn't the case for XML. XML's DTDs are not published by the W3C; it is up to the Web developer to create the DTD. Because of this, Web developers don't have to force data to fit into existing tags, but instead create tags to support existing data. This new model allows Web developers to extend the rules of XML when needed.

Index
(Item numbers refer to sections of the book)

Symbols
"0"
    3.10, 3.12, 3.18,
    4.3, 4.6, 4.24,
    5.3, 5.7, 5.8, 5.9

"0.5"
    3.18,
    4.3, 4.4, 4.5, 4.6

"1"
    3.10, 3.12, 3.18,
    4.3, 4.4, 4.5, 4.6, 4.7, 4.8, 4.9, 4.10, 4.11, 4.12, 4.13,
    5.3, 5.7, 5.8, 5.9

.NET
    6.14,

A

Artificial Neural Network(s) -ANN(s), Network
    Preface,
    1.1, 1.2, 1.3, 1.4, 1.5, 1.6, 1.7, 1.8, 1.10, 1.11, 1.12,
    2.5, 2.7, 2.8, 2.9, 2.10, 2.12, 2.13, 2.15, 2.16,
    3.3, 3.5, 3.7, 3.8, 3.9, 3.10, 3.11, 3.12, 3.16, 3.17, 3.18, 3.19, 3.22, 3.23,
                     3.25, 3.26, 3.27, 3.28, 3.30, 3.32,
    4.1, 4.2, 4.3, 4.4, 4.5, 4.6, 4.9, 4.13, 4.14, 4.15, 4.16, 4.17, 4.18, 4.24,
                     4.25,
    5.1, 5.2, 5.3, 5.4, 5.5, 5.9, 5.10, 5.11, 5.12, 5.13, 5.15, 5.16,
    7.1, 7.2, 7.3

... Categories
    1.6

... FFA
    1.2, 1.3, 1.4, 1.5, 1.6, 1.7,
    2.1, 2.7, 2.8, 2.9, 2.12, 2.13, 2.16,
    3.7, 3.9, 3.10, 3.19, 3.22, 3.23, 3.25, 3.30, 3.32,
    4.1, 4.2, 4.4, 4.9, 4.13, 4.14, 4.15, 4.17, 4.18, 4.24, 4.25,
    5.2, 5.5, 5.8, 5.12, 5.13, 5.15, 5.16,
    7.1, 7.2, 7.3

... Hardware/Software design
    1.4, 1.10, 1.12,
    2.2, 2.3, 2.8, 1.13, 2.16,

3.3, 3.6, 3.32,
4.2, 4.4, 4.17, 4.18, 4.24,
5.1, 5.2, 5.3, 5.4, 5.5, 5.6, 5.11, 5.12, 5.13, 5.15, 5.16,
7.2, 7.3

... Learning/Training
Preface,
1.1, 1.2, 1.3, 1.4, 1.5, 1.6, 1.7, 1.8, 1.9, 1.10, 1.11, 1.12,
2.2, 2.3, 2.4, 2.7, 2.8, 2.9, 2.10, 2.12,
3.1, 3.3, 3.5, 3.7, 3.8, 3.10, 3.11, 3.12, 3.13, 3.14, 3.17, 3.18, 3.19, 3.22,
3.23, 3.25, 3.30, 3.31, 3.323.18, 3.31,
4.1, 4.2, 4.3, 4.4, 4.5, 4.16, 4.17, 4.24, 4.25,
5.1, 5.2, 5.3, 5.4, 5.10, 5.11, 5.12, 5.13, 5.16, 5.17,
7.1, 7.2, 7.3

... Sigmoid
1.2, 1,7,
3.23,
5.2, 5.32, 5.42, 5.52, 5.62, 5.72, 5.92, 5.102, 5.152, 5.16,
7.2

... Weight(s)
Preface,
1.2, 1.3, 1.4, 1.7, 1.8, 1.9, 1.11,
2.8, 2.9, 2.13,
3.8, 3.11, 3.15, 3.19, 3.22, 3.29,
4.1, 4.2, 4.6, 4.9, 4.15, 4.18, 4.19, 4.20, 4.21, 4.22, 4.23, 4.24, 4.25,
5.2, 5.4, 5.5, 5.6, 5.7, 5.8, 5.9, 5.10, 5.11, 5.12, 5.14, 5.15,
7.2, 7.3

B

Back Propagation
1.7, 1.8,
2.9,
3.8, 3.9, 3.10,
4.16,
5.3,
7.1, 7.2

C

Clinical Differential Diagnosis Methodology (CDDM)
3.4, 3.7, 3.15, 3.16, 3.17, 3.19, 3.22, 3.25, 3.29, 3.31,
5.5

COM
6.6, 6.7, 6.8, 6.9, 6.10, 6.11, 6.12, 6.13,
ApII.1,
ApIII.1, ApIII.2

D

DCOM
  6.13,
  ApIII.1, ApIII.2
Decision Support System(s) -DSS(s), System(s)
  Preface,
  1.10,
  2.1, 2.2, 2.3, 2.4, 2.5, 2.6, 2.7, 2.8, 2.9, 2.10, 2.11, 2.12, 2.13, 2.15,
  3.1, 3.2, 3.3, 3.4, 3.5, 3.13, 3.14, 3.16, 3.19,
  4.3, 4.4, 4.5, 4.6, 4.14, 4.15, 4.16, 4.25,
  5.1, 5.2, 5.3, 5.4, 5.5, 5.6, 5.7, 5.9, 5.10, 5.12, 5.13, 5.15, 5.16,
  7.1, 7.3
... Layer
  2.11, 2.12, 2.13
  3.8, 3.9, 3.10, 3.11, 3.19, 3.20, 3.21, 3.22, 3.23, 3.25, 3.26, 3.27, 3.28,
      3.30,
  5.4, 5.15,
  7.1
... Hidden Layer
  3.8, 3.9, 3.10, 3.11, 3.22,
  5.4
... Level
  2.11, 2.12, 2.13,
  3.15, 3.19, 3.20, 3.21, 3.22, 3.30
Disease(s)
  4.5,
  5.3, 5.4, 5.5,
  7.3
... Haematologic
  3.30,
  5.3, 5.4, 5.5,
  7.2
... Pulmonary
  0.1,
  3.16, 3.17, 3.18, 3.20, 3.22, 3.24,
  5.3, 5.4, 5.5,
  7.2
... Category(ies) of
  3.7, 3.15, 3.16, 3.18, 3.20, 3.21, 3.22, 3.23, 3.24, 3.30,
  4.5
... Finding(s)
  3.2, 3.3, 3.4, 3.5, 3.6, 3.7, 3.8, 3.9, 3.10, 3.11, 3.12, 3.13, 3.14, 3.15,
      3.16, 3.17, 3.18, 3.21, 3.22, 3.23, 3.24, 3.25, 3.29, 3.30,
  4.4, 4.5, 4.6, 4.15, 4.25,
  5.3, 5.4

E

Expert System(s)
2.9
4.16

F

FFA-ANN
see ANN > FFA
Findings of Diseases
see Diseases > Findings

G

Generation of Learning Patterns
see Learning Patterns > Generation

H

Haematologic Diseases
see Diseases > Haematologic
Haematology
3.1, 3.5, 3.29, 3.30, 3.31,
4.16,
5.16
Hardware design of ANN
see ANN > Hardware
Hidden Layer
see DSS > Hidden Layer
Hidden Neurons
see Neurons > Hidden
Hidden Slabs
see Slabs > Hidden

L

Layer of Decision Support System
see DSS > Layer
Learning of ANNs
see ANN > Learning
Learning Pattern(s), Pattern(s)
0.1, 0.2,
1.3, 1.4, 1.5, 1.7, 1.8, 1.9, 1.10, 1.11, 1.12,
2.2, 2.3, 2.7, 2.8, 2.9, 2.10, 2.12, 2.13, 2.15
3.1, 3.2, 3.5, 3.7, 3.8, 3.9, 3.10, 3.11, 3.12, 3.14, 3.16, 3.18, 3.19, 3.22,
3.23, 3.25, 3.29, 3.30, 3.31, 3.32,
4.1, 4.2, 4.3, 4.4, 4.5, 4.6, 4.9, 4.13, 4.14, 4.15, 4.16, 4.17, 4.18, 4.25,
5.2, 5.3, 5.4, 5.10, 5.13,
7.1, 7.2, 7.3

... Generation
> 4.5
... Logical level of input data
> 1.8,
> 3.18,
> 4.3, 4.4, 4.5, 4.6, 4.7, 4.8, 4.9, 4.10, 4.11, 4.12, 4.13, 4.25,
> 5.3, 5.7
... Pseudo-input(s)
> 3.19,
> 4.5, 4.6, 4.7, 4.8, 4.9, 4.12, 4.15,
> 7.2

Level of Decision Support System
> see DSS > Level

Logical level of input data
> see Learning Patterns > Logical level of input data

M

Medical Decision Support System(s) -MDSS(s), Medical System
> 3.1, 3.2, 3.3, 3.4, 3.5, 3.6, 3.7, 3.8, 3.9, 3.12, 3.13, 3.15, 3.16, 3.17,
> 3.19, 3.22, 3.23, 3.25, 3.29, 3.30, 3.31,
> 4.3, 4.4, 4.5,
> 5.1, 5.2, 5.3, 5.4, 5.5, 5.9, 5.13,
> 7.2, 7.3,
> ApxI.1

N

Neuron(s)
> 1.1, 1.2, 1.3, 1.4, 1.5, 1.7, 1.8, 1.9, 1.11,
> 2.8, 2.12, 2.13, 2.15, 2.16,
> 3.8, 3.9, 3.10, 3.11, 3.19, 3.23, 3.25, 3.26, 3.27, 3.28, 3.29,
> 4.1, 4.2, 4.15, 4.16, 4.17, 4.18, 4.19, 4.20, 4.21, 4.22, 4.23, 4.25,
> 5.1, 5.2, 5.5, 5.6, 5.7, 5.8, 5.9, 5.12, 5.13, 5.14, 5.15, 5.16,
> 7.2, 7.3

... Hidden
> 1.3, 1.4, 1.7, 1.8,
> 2.4,
> 3.29,
> 4.2, 4.15, 4.16, 4.17, 4.18, 4.19, 4.20, 4.21, 4.22, 4.23, 4.25,
> 7.2

P

Pseudo-input(s)
> see Learning Patterns > Pseudo-input(s)

Pulmonary Diseases
> see Diseases > Pulmonary

Pulmonology
> 1.1,
> 3.25,
> 4.16,
> 5.16

S

Sigmoid Function
> see ANN > Sigmoid

Slab(s)
> 1.3, 1.4, 1.5, 1.7, 1.9,
> 2.8, 2.9, 2.11, 2.12, 2.15, 2.16,
> 3.20, 3.22, 3.23, 3.30,
> 4.1, 4.2, 4.15, 4.16, 4.17, 4.25,
> 5.9,
> 7.2

… Hidden
> 1.3, 1.4, 1.5, 1.7, 1.9,
> 2.15,
> 3.23,
> 4.1, 4.2, 4.15, 4.16, 4.17, 4.25,
> 7.2

Software design of ANN
> see ANN > Software

Synapses
> 1.1, 1.3, 1.8,
> 2.8, 2.9, 2.12,
> 3.9, 3.23, 3.25, 3.26, 3.27, 3.28,
> 4.15, 4.16, 4.18, 4.19, 4.20, 4.21, 4.22, 4.23, 4.24, 4.25,
> 5.2, 5.4, 5.5, 5.9, 5.10, 5.11, 5.12,
> 7.2

T

Tele-Medicine
> Preface,
> 6.2, 6.3, 6.13, 6.14

Tele-Working
> Preface,
> 6.1, 6.3

Tele-Working Platform
> Preface,
> 6.1, 6.2, 6.14,
> 7.2

Training of ANNs
> see ANN > Training

W

Weights of ANN
   see ANN > Weights

Printed in the United Kingdom
by Lightning Source UK Ltd.
102363UKS00001B/145-210